CORE COLLECTION OF MEDICAL BOOKS AND JOURNALS 2001

Fourth Edition

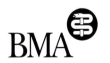

BMA

Compiled by
Howard Hague

Medical Information Working Party, London

i

Compiler:
Howard Hague MA, ALA
Library, Charing Cross Campus
Imperial College of Science, Technology
and Medicine
Reynolds Building
St Dunstan's Road
London W6 8RP

Chairman of MIWP:
Paul Harwood
Swets Blackwell
32 Blacklands Way
Abingdon Business Park
Abingdon
Oxon OX14 1SX

Contact for INFAH
(Information Focus for Allied Health):
Anna Sewerniak
Senior Information Officer
Chartered Society of Physiotherapy
14 Bedford Row
London WC1R 4ED

MEDICAL INFORMATION
WORKING PARTY

Melanie Brocklehurst
Information Service
Wellcome Library
183 Euston Road
London NW1 2BE

Gordon Brooks MB chB, PhD
Head of Knowledge Support
EMIS
Fort Fareham Business Park
Newgate Lane
Fareham PO14 1AH

Maureen Forrest
John Radcliffe Hospital
Cairns Library
Headington
Oxford OX3 9DU

Sue Gregory
Blackwell's Medical Bookshop
Queens Medical Centre
Clifton Boulevard
Nottingham NG7 2UH

Howard Hague
Library, Charing Cross Campus
Imperial College of Science, Technology
and Medicine
Reynolds Building
St Dunstan's Road
London W6 8RP

Paul Harwood
Swets Blackwell
32 Blacklands Way
Abingdon Business Park
Abingdon
Oxon OX14 1SX

Annette Herholdt
John Wiley & Sons Ltd
4th Floor, International House
7 High Street
Ealing
London W5 5DB

Richard Jones
BMA Library
BMA House
Tavistock Square
London WC1H 9JP

Peter Lawson
Karger
58 Grove Hill Road
Tunbridge Wells
Kent TN1 1SP

David Morgan
Cambridge Medical Books
Units 8/9 Hurlingham Business Park
Sulivan Road
London SW6 3DU

Cath Mundell
Oxford University Press
Great Clarendon Street
Oxford OX2 6DP

Tony Roche
Everetts
Unit 8
Hurlingham Business Park
Sulivan Road
London SW6 3DU

Rollo Turner
Association of Subscription Agents & Intermediaries
10 Lime Avenue
High Wycombe
Buckinghamshire HP11 1DP

For further copies of the Core Collection contact:
Alex Osborne
Cambridge Medical Books
Units 8/9 Hurlingham Business Park
Sulivan Road
London SW6 3DU

The gateway to a world of information

In a changing world, vision, experience and reliability are the qualities you value in a partner. Whether it be the management of your subscriptions or the delivery of an article to your desktop, Swets Blackwell provides quality services to libraries and information centres all over the world.

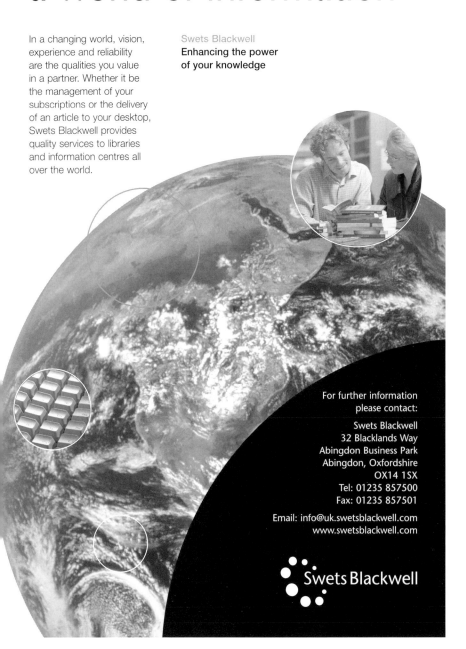

CONTENTS

PREFACE

The Medical Information Working Party is delighted to present the 4th edition of the Core Collection of Medical Books and Journals. First published in 1992, the Core Collection has established itself as a reliable acquisition guide for the small to medium sized library in a hospital or comparable medical institute, and provides a useful counterbalance to the 'Brandon/Hill' list which appears in the Bulletin of the Medical Library Association.

The Core Collection will never lay claim to being a definitive list of titles, but a recommended selection of the essential material that every medical library should stock. In the UK, it has become an established selection tool as well as a means of supporting bids for additional funding. In some cases, it has been used as an accreditation standard for libraries serving postgraduate medical education.

The subject coverage of the 4th edition has once again been broadened to include: Communication Skills, and Clinical Governance (the latter within Health Administration), and the number of titles included has been increased to over 1580.

It would cost £86,280 to purchase all of the books and £85,768 to subscribe to all of the journals in this core list. This is a total cost of £172,048 (These totals are based on prices known at the time of going to press). This compares with a total cost of £125,253 for the books and journals in the 1997 list.

The Medical Information Working Party is once again indebted to Howard Hague, Assistant Librarian at Imperial College of Science, Technology and Medicine, for compiling this list, and to Melanie Brocklehurst and Richard Jones for editing and proof-reading it. Howard's considerable experience as a professional librarian and the lessons learnt from compiling the previous three editions have all gone into making this 4th edition the most comprehensive of all. It stands as a quality publication in all respects. Howard would be the first to acknowledge the help he has received in a variety of different areas from: Graeme Barber; Clare Burnham; John Eyres; Debbie Heatlie; Liz James; Richard Jones; Richard Peacock; Anna Sewerniak; Rachel Shipton; Neroli Wolland.

If you have used the Core Collection before, I hope you find the latest edition as useful as the previous editions. If you are new to it, then I hope it will become a standard reference work on your personal library shelf.

Paul Harwood
Chair, Medical Information Working Party

ACCIDENT & EMERGENCY MEDICINE

Brown, A.F.T.
Accident and emergency
Butterworth-Heinemann 380pp 3e. Paperback 1996
0-7506-2233-4   £18.99

Capehorn, D.
Handbook of paediatric accident and emergency medicine
Bailliere Tindall 432pp 1998
0-7020-2168-7   £21.95

Colquhoun, M.C.
ABC of resuscitation
BMJ Books 104pp 4e. Paperback 1999
0-7279-1190-2   £14.95

Currie, D.
The management of head injuries
Oxford UP 206pp 2e. Paperback 2000
0-19-263078-4   £26.95

Driscoll, P.
Trauma care: beyond the resuscitation room
BMJ Books 322pp 1998
0-7279-0933-9   £135.00

Ellis, B. M.
Hamilton Bailey's Emergency Surgery
Butterworth-Heinemann 13e. Hardback 2000
0-7506-4253-X   £120.00

Ferguson, D.G.
Colour guide: accident and emergency medicine
Churchill Livingstone 160pp 2e. Paperback 1998
0-443-06029-0   £11.95

Greaves, I.
Practical accident and emergency medicine
Butterworth-Heinemann 384pp 2000
0-7506-3421-9   £35.00

Guly, U.
Acute medical emergencies
Oxford UP 232pp 1996
0-19-262558-6   £16.95

Higginson, I.
What to do in a paediatric emergency
BMJ Books 60pp 1996
0-7279-1032-9   £13.95

Hodgetts, T.
Evidence-based pre-hospital care
Oxford UP 512pp Plastic-reinforced paper 2001
0-19-262917-4   £19.95

Monson, J.
Surgical emergencies
Blackwell Science UK 448pp Hardback 1999
0-632-05047-0   £75.00

Morton, R.J.
Accidents and emergencies in children
Oxford UP 282pp 2e. 1996
0-19-262720-1 Hardback   £29.95
0-19-262719-8 Paperback   £16.95

Moulton, C.
Lecture notes on emergency medicine
Blackwell Science UK 357pp Paperback 1999
0-632-02766-5   £19.95

Nicholson, D.
ABC of emergency radiology
BMJ Books 100pp 1995
0-7279-0832-4   £17.95

Ramrakha, P.S.
Oxford handbook of acute medicine
Oxford UP 892pp Paperback 1997
0-19-262682-5   £16.95

Skinner, D.
ABC of major trauma
BMJ Books 168pp 3e. Paperback 1999
0-7279-1378-6   £18.95

Skinner, D.V.
Cambridge textbook of accident and emergency medicine
Cambridge UP 1285pp Hardback 1997
0-521-43379-7   £160.00

Skinner, D.V.
Cardiopulmonary resuscitation
Oxford UP 232pp 2e. Paperback 1996
0-19-262693-0   £16.95

Sprigings, D.C.
Acute medicine
Blackwell Science UK 440pp 2e.
Paperback 1995
0-632-03652-4   £18.50

Unwin, A.
Emergency orthopaedics & trauma
Butterworth-Heinemann 288pp 1995
0-7506-2034-X   £25.00

Wardrope, J.
The management of wounds and burns
Oxford UP 256pp 2e.1999
0-19-262999-9   £24.95

Wardrope, J.
Musculo-skeletal problems in emergency medicine
Oxford UP 348pp 1998
0-19-262863-1 Hardback   £49.50
0-19-262862-3 Paperback   £24.95

Webb, L.
Eye emergencies Butterworth-Heinemann
196pp Paperback 1995
0-7506-2015-3   £21.50

Wyatt, J.P.
Oxford handbook of accident and emergency medicine
Oxford UP 800pp 1999
0-19-262751-1 £18.95

AIDS & HIV
(See also Sexually transmitted diseases)

Adler, M.W.
ABC of AIDS
BMJ Books 100pp Paperback 1997
0-7279-1137-6 £17.95

Alcorn, K.
HIV and AIDS treatment directory
NAM Publications 480pp Paperback 1999
1-898397-47-3 £57.50

Bennett, R.
HIV and AIDS, testing, screening, and confidentiality
Clarendon Press 302pp Hardback 1999
0-19-823801-0 £35.00

Berridge, V.
AIDS in the UK
Oxford UP 404pp 1996
0-19-820472-8 Hardback £50.00
0-19-820473-6 Paperback £14.99

Crowe, S.
Management of the HIV infected patient
Isis Medical Media 512pp 2e. Hardback 2000
1-901865-28-2 £95.00

De Vita Jr, V.T.
AIDS
Lippincott-Raven 768pp 4e. Hardback 1997
0-397-51538-3 £73.00

Merigan, T.C.
Textbook of AIDS medicine
Williams and Wilkins 1064pp 2e. Hardback 1998
0-683-30216-7 £105.00

Palfreeman, A.
Drugs in HIV and AIDS
John Wiley 124pp 2e. Paperback 1998
0-471-97063-8 £17.99

Penneys, N.S.
Skin manifestations of AIDS
Martin Dunitz 264pp 2e. Hardback 1995
1-85317-242-1 £49.95

Pizzo, P.A.
Pediatric AIDS
Williams and Wilkins 1000pp 3e. 1999
0-683-30399-6 £69.00

Sande, M.A.
The medical management of AIDS
W.B. Saunders 636pp 6e. Paperback 1999
0-7216-8102-6 £55.00

Schoub, B.D.
AIDS and HIV in Perspective
Cambridge UP 296pp Paperback 1999
0-521-62766-4 Paperback £17.95
0-521-62150-X Hardback £50.00

ANAESTHESIA & INTENSIVE CARE

Adams, A.P.
Emergency anaesthesia
Arnold 448pp 2e. Paperback 1998
0-340-69219-7 £34.99

Aitkenhead, A.R.
Textbook of anaesthesia
Churchill Livingstone 788pp 3e. Paperback 1996
0-443-05056-2 £45.00

Anderson, I.
Care of the critically ill surgical patient
Arnold 224pp 1999
0-340-70092-0 £32.50

Bion, J.F.
Intensive care medicine
BMJ Books 456pp 1999
0-7279-1076-0 £45.00

Calvey, T.N.
Principles and practice of pharmacology for anaesthetists
Blackwell Science UK 608pp 3e. Hardback 1996
0-632-04156-0 £79.50

Campbell, S.D.
Norris & Campbell's anaesthetics, resuscitation and intensive care
Churchill Livingstone 272pp 8e. Paperback 1996
0-443-04886-X £19.95

Craft, T.
Key topics in critical care
Bios Scientific 288pp Paperback1999
1-85996-286-6 £19.95

Craft, T.M.
Key topics in anaesthesia
Bios Scientific 360pp 2e. Paperback 1995
1-85996-075-8 £21.95

Cruickshank, S.
Mathematics and statistics in anaesthesia
Oxford UP 268pp 1998
0-19-262313-3 Hardback £49.50
0-19-262312-5 Paperback £24.95

Davis, P.D.
Basic physics and measurement in anaesthesia
Butterworth-Heinemann 380pp Paperback 1995
0-7506-1713-6 £35.00

Duncan, A.
Paediatric intensive care
BMJ Books 287pp Paperback 1998
0-7279-1073-6 £30.00

Ellis, H.
Anatomy for anaesthetists
Blackwell Science UK 384pp 7e. Hardback 1996
0-86542-721-6 £62.50

Gothard, J.
Essentials of cardiac and thoracic anaesthesia
Butterworth-Heinemann 196pp Paperback 1999
0-7506-2033-1 £22.50

Gwinnutt, C.L.
Clinical anaesthesia
Blackwell Science UK 400pp Paperback 1996
0-86542-749-6 £18.50

Gwinnutt, C.L.
Lecture notes on clinical anaesthesia
Blackwell Science USA 224pp 5e. Paperback 1997
0-86542-656-2 £14.95

Hatch, D.J.
Textbook of paediatric anaesthesia
Arnold 512pp 2e. Hardback 1999
0-340-71942-7 £65.00

Healy, T.E.J.
Aids to anaesthesia
Churchill Livingstone 224pp 2e. Paperback 1999
0-443-04233-0 £14.95

Healy, T.E.J.
Wylie and Churchill-Davidson's A practice of anaesthesia
Arnold 1560pp 6e. Hardback 1995
0-340-55309-X £145.00

Hinds, C.J.
Intensive care
W B Saunders 576pp 2e. Paperback 1996
0-7020-1541-5 £34.95

Holdcroft, A.
Principles and practice of obstetric anaesthesia
Blackwell Science USA 384pp Hardback 1999
0-86542-828-X £75.00

Illingworth, K.A.
Anaesthesia and analgesia in emergency medicine
Oxford UP 406pp Paperback 1998
0-19-262909-3 Hardback £45.00
0-19-262908-5 Paperback £24.95

Lumb, A.
Nunn's applied respiratory physiology
Butterworth-Heinemann 448pp 5e. Hardback 1999
0-7506-3107-4 £59.50

Mather, S.J.
A handbook of paediatric anaesthesia
Oxford UP 288pp 2e. Hardback 1996
0-19-262714-7 £27.50

Miller, R.D.
Anesthesia
2 vols & CD-ROM Churchill Livingstone 3168pp 5e.
Hardback 1999
0-443-07988-9 £175.00

Moyle, J.T.B.
Ward's anaesthetic equipment
W B Saunders 399pp 4e. Hardback 1998
0-7020-2169-5 £45.00

Oh, T.E.
Intensive care manual
Butterworth-Heinemann 1032pp 4e. Paperback 1997
0-7506-2358-6 £45.00

Pinnock, C.
Fundamentals of anaesthesia
Greenwich Medical 750pp Paperback 1999
1-900151-61-8 £55.00

Prys-Roberts, C.
International practice of anaesthesia
2 vols Butterworth-Heinemann 2600pp Hardback 1996
0-7506-0240-6 £275.00

Rushman, G.B.
Lee's synopsis of anaesthesia
Butterworth-Heinemann 560pp 12e. Paperback 1999
0-7506-3247-X £27.50

Sasada, M.
Drugs in anaesthesia and intensive care
Oxford UP 414pp 2e. Plastic-reinforced paper 1997
0-19-262872-0 £19.95

Singer, M.
ABC of intensive care
BMJ Books 72pp 1999
0-7279-1436-7 £15.95

Singer, M.
Oxford handbook of critical care
Oxford UP 560pp 1997
0-19-262542-X £19.95

Vickers, M.D.
Drugs in anaesthetic and intensive care practice
Butterworth-Heinemann 496pp Hardback 1999
0-7506-3727-7 £55.00

Vickers, M.D.
Medicine for anaesthetists
Blackwell Science USA 408pp 4e. Hardback 1999
0-86542-637-6 £79.50

Webb, A.
Oxford textbook of critical care
Oxford UP 1458pp Hardback 1999
0-19-262737-6 £165.00

Yentis, S.
FRCA survival guide
Butterworth-Heinemann 128pp Paperback 1998
0-7506-3718-8 £14.99

ANATOMY, HISTOLOGY & EMBRYOLOGY

Abrahams, P.H.
McMinn's colour atlas of human anatomy
Mosby 368pp 4e. 1998
0-7234-2641-4 Hardback £42.95
0-7234-2772-0 Paperback £32.95

Agur, A.M.R.
Grant's atlas of anatomy
Williams and Wilkins 704pp 10e. Paperback 1999
0-683-30264-7 £29.95

Bancroft, J.D.
Theory and practice of histological techniques
Churchill Livingstone 766pp 4e. Hardback 1995
0-443-04760-X £99.95

Ellis, H.
Clinical anatomy
Blackwell Science UK 464pp 9e. Paperback 1997
0-86542-882-4 £29.95

Eroschenko, V.P.
Di Fiore's atlas of histology with clinical correlations
Lippincott, Williams and Wilkins 9e. Paperback 2000
0-683-30749-5 £27.95

Gosling, J.A.
Human anatomy: color atlas and text
Mosby 112pp 3e. Paperback 1996
0-7234-2657-0 £28.95

Kiernan, J.A.
Barr's The Human Nervous System
Williams and Wilkins 518pp 7e. Paperback with diskette 1998
0-397-58431-8 £23.50

Lumley, J.S.P.
Essential anatomy - and some clinical applications
Churchill Livingstone 600pp 5e. Paperback 1995
0-443-04808-8 £19.95

Moore, K.
Clinically oriented anatomy
Williams and Wilkins 1200pp 4e. Paperback 1999
0-683-06141-0 £35.00

Moore, K.L.
The developing human
W B Saunders 563pp 6e. Paperback 1998
0-7216-6974-3 £26.95

Sadler, T.
Langman's medical embryology
Williams and Wilkins 500pp 8e.Paperback 2000
0-683-30650-2 £23.95

Sinnatamby, C.S.
Last's anatomy
Churchill Livingstone 552pp 10e. Paperback 1999
0-443-05611-0 £35.00

Snell, R.S.
Clinical anatomy for medical students
Lippincott, Williams and Wilkins 6e. Paperback 2000
0-7817-1574-1 £29.95

Stevens, A.
Human histology
Mosby 416pp 2e. Paperback 1996
0-7234-2485-3 £26.95

Williams, P.L.
Gray's anatomy
Churchill Livingstone 38e. 1995
0-443-04560-7 Hardback £140.00
0-443-06390-7 CD-ROM £199.95

Young, B.
Wheater's functional histology
Churchill Livingstone 416pp 4e. Paperback 2000
0-443-05612-9 £34.95

BIOCHEMISTRY & CELL BIOLOGY

Alberts, B.
Essential cell biology
Garland Publishing 630pp Paperback 1998
0-8153-2971-7 £26.95

Campbell, P.N.
Biochemistry illustrated
Churchill Livingstone 240pp 4e. Paperback 2000
0-443-06217-X £24.95

Devlin, T.M.
Textbook of biochemistry with clinical correlations
John Wiley 1214pp 4e. Hardback with CD-ROM 1997
0-471-15451-2 £32.50

Gaw, A.
Clinical biochemistry
Churchill Livingstone176pp 2e. Paperback 1999
0-443-06183-1 £19.95

Gillham, B.
Wills' biochemical basis of medicine
Butterworth-Heinemann 544pp 3e. Paperback 1997
0-7506-2013-7 £32.50

Goodman, S.R.
Medical cell biology
Williams and Wilkins 320pp 2e. Mixed-media
pack 1998
0-397-58427-X   £25.00

Lodish, H.
Molecular cell biology
W H Freeman 1296pp 4e. With CD-ROM 1999
0-7167-3706-X   £34.95

Montgomery, R.
Biochemistry: a case oriented approach
Mosby 700pp 6e. Paperback 1996
0-8151-6483-1   £38.95

Murray, R.K.
Harper's biochemistry
Appleton and Lange 960pp 25e. Paperback 2000
0-8385-3684-0   £28.99

Nelson, D.L.
Lehninger: Principles of biochemistry
Worth Publishers 3e. 2000
1-57259-931-6   £34.95

Stryer, L.
Biochemistry
W H Freeman 1064pp 4e. Hardback 1995
0-7167-2009-4   £32.95

Trent, R.J.A.
Molecular medicine
Churchill Livingstone241pp 2e. Paperback 1997
0-443-05366-9   £19.95

Williams, D.
Scientific foundations of biochemistry in clinical practice
Butterworth-Heinemann 800pp 2e. Paperback 1998
0-7506-4221-1   £65.00

CARDIOLOGY

Alexander, R.W.
Hurst's the heart
McGraw-Hill USA 2480pp 9e. Hardback 1998
0-07-057717-X   £97.99

Beevers, D.G.
Hypertension in practice
Martin Dunitz 256pp 3e. Hardback 1999
1-85317-591-9   £49.95

Belch, J.J.F.
Color atlas of peripheral vascular diseases
Mosby 138pp 2e. Hardback 1996
0-7234-2074-2   £55.00

Bennett, D.H.
Cardiac arrhythmias
Butterworth-Heinemann 245pp 5e. Paperback 1997
0-7506-3369-7   £25.00

Braunwald, E.
Essential atlas of heart diseases
Appleton and Lange 336pp 1997
0-8385-2215-7   £96.99

Braunwald, E.
Heart disease
W B Saunders 2143pp 5e. Hardback 1997
0-7216-5666-8 (In 1 vol)   £99.00
0-7216-5663-3 (In 2 vols)   £110.00

Chien, K.R.
Molecular basis of heart disease
W B Saunders 590pp 1999
0-7216-6401-6   £95.00

Fowler, N.O.
Physical signs in cardiology
Mosby 240pp 1999
0-7234-3105-1   £19.95

Goldberger, A.L.
Clinical electrocardiography
Mosby 384pp 6e. Paperback 1999
0-3230-0252-8   £29.95

Gray, H.
Lecture notes on cardiology
Blackwell Science UK 288pp 4e. Paperback 2001
0-86542-864-6   £12.95

Hampton, J.R.
The ECG in practice
Churchill Livingstone320pp 3e. Paperback 1997
0-443-05680-3   £15.95

Hampton, J.R.
The ECG made easy
Churchill Livingstone129pp 5e. Paperback 1997
0-443-05681-1   £9.95

Houghton, A.R.
Making sense of the ECG
Arnold 288pp 1997
0-340-67657-4   £15.99

Izzo Jr, J.L.
Hypertension primer: the essentials of high blood pressure
Williams and Wilkins 496pp 2e. Paperback 1999
0-683-30706-1   £19.00

Jackson, G.
Angina - pocketbook
Martin Dunitz 80pp 3e. Paperback 2000
1-85317-626-5   £9.95

Jackson, G.
Difficult cardiology
Martin Dunitz 300pp 3e. 1997
1-85317-406-8   £65.00

Julian, D.G.
Cardiology
W B Saunders 440pp 7e. Paperback 1998
0-7020-2211-X £19.95

Julian, D.G.
Diseases of the heart
W B Saunders Co 1617pp 2e. Hardback 1996
0-7020-1756-6 £112.00

Julian, D.G.
Women and heart disease
Martin Dunitz 432pp 1997
1-85317-287-1 £75.00

Kern, M.J.
The cardiac catheterization handbook
Mosby 640pp 3e. Spiral bound 1994
0-8151-2614-X £34.95

Khan, M.G.
Cardiac drug therapy
W B Saunders 456pp 5e. Paperback 1999
0-7020-2479-1 £22.95

Lip, G.
Key topics in cardiovascular medicine
Bios Scientific 208pp 1998
1-85996-101-0 £18.95

Matthews, L.R.
Cardiopulmonary anatomy and physiology
Lippincott-Raven 336pp 1996
0-397-54954-7 £19.75

O'Brien, E.
ABC of hypertension
BMJ Books 112pp 4e. Paperback 2000
0-7279-1522-3 £15.00

Otto, C.M.
Valvular heart disease
W B Saunders 480pp 1999
0-7216-7139-X £85.00

Shapiro, L.M.
Color atlas of heart failure
Mosby 160pp Hardback 1995
0-7234-2023-8 £55.00

Sutton, G.C.
Clinical cardiology: an illustrated text
Chapman and Hall 448pp Hardback 1998
0-412-78310-X £89.00

Swanton, R.H.
Pocket consultant: cardiology
Blackwell Science UK 568pp 4e. Paperback 1997
0-632-04839-5 £19.95

Thompson, D.R.
Cardiac rehabilitation guidelines and audit standards
Royal College of Physicians 130pp 1997
1-86016-048-4 £12.50

Timmis, A.
Diagnosis in color: cardiology
Mosby 328pp 1997
0-7234-2551-5 £21.95

Timmis, A.D.
Essential cardiology
Blackwell Science UK 392pp Paperback 1997
0-632-04843-3 £24.95

Topol, E.J.
Textbook of cardiovascular medicine
Lippincott 2760pp 1998
0-397-51592-8 £83.25

Topol, E.J.
Textbook of interventional cardiology
W B Saunders 848pp 3e. Hardback 1999
0-7216-7676-6 £115.00

Volta, S.D.
Cardiology
McGraw-Hill 834pp Paperback 1999
0-07-709518-9 £34.99

Wagner, G.S.
Marriott's practical electrocardiography
Lippincott, Williams and Wilkins 450pp 10e. 2000
0-683-30746-0 £26.50

Walsh, C.A.
Practical echocardiography
Greenwich Medical 228pp 1999
1-900151-86-3 £32.50

Yusuf, S.
Evidence based cardiology
BMJ Books 1134pp Hardback 1998
0-7279-1171-6 £130.00

COMMUNICATION SKILLS

British Medical Association
Communication skills and continuing professional development
BMJ Books 16pp Paperback 1998
0-7279-1390-5 £5.00

Burnard, P.
Effective communication skills for health professionals
Stanley Thornes 271pp 2e. Paperback 1997
0-7487-3312-4 £17.50

Enelow, A.J.
Interviewing and patient care
Oxford UP Inc 224pp 4e. 1996
0-19-506443-7 Hardback £31.50
0-19-506444-5 Paperback £17.95

Fielding, R.
Clinical communication skills
Hong Kong Uni Press 352pp 1995
962-209-371-X £19.95

Hind, C.R.K.
Communication skills in medicine
BMJ Books 161pp Paperback 1997
0-7279-1152-X £15.95

Kurtz, S.
Teaching and learning communication skills in medicine
Radcliffe Medical 272pp Hardback 1998
1-85775-273-2 £35.00

Lloyd, M.
Communication skills for medicine
Churchill Livingstone 190pp Paperback 1996
0-443-05168-2 £17.95

Maguire, P.
Communication skills for doctors
Arnold 192pp Paperback 2000
0-340-66309-X £12.99

Myerscough, P.R.
Talking with patients
Oxford UP 258pp 3e. Paperback 1996
0-19-262570-5 £19.95

Silverman, J.
Skills for communicating with patients
Radcliffe Medical 200pp 1997
1-85775-189-2 £18.95

Tate, P.
The doctor's communication handbook
Radcliffe Medical 152pp 2e. Paperback 1997
1-85775-256-2 £17.95

COMMUNITY CARE
(See also Geriatric Medicine)

Barnes, M.
Unequal partners: user groups and community care
The Policy Press 120pp Paperback 1999
1-86134-056-7 £13.99

Barnes, M.
Care, communities and citizens
Longman Higher Education 212pp Paperback 1997
0-582-25129-X £19.99

Bartlett, P.
Outside the walls of the asylum
Athlone Press 260pp Paperback 1999
0-485-12147-6 £16.99

Beales, D.
Community care of older people
Radcliffe Medical 224pp Paperback 1997
1-85775-032-2 £18.95

Bornat, J.
Community care
Macmillan Press 368pp 2e. 1997
0-333-69846-0 Hardback £47.50
0-333-69847-9 Paperback £15.99

Carnell, J.
Community practitioners and health visitors handbook
Radcliffe Medical 152pp Paperback 1999
1-85775-371-2 £13.95

Dimond, B.
Legal aspects of care in the community
Macmillan Press 672pp 1996
0-333-53819-6 Hardback £55.00
0-333-53820-X Paperback £23.50

Jack, R.
Residential versus community care
Macmillan Press 240pp Paperback 1998
0-333-66518-X £15.99

Leff, J.
Care in the community
John Wiley 230pp 1997
0-471-96981-8 Hardback £55.00
0-471-96982-6 Paperback £16.99

Lewis, J.
Implementing the new community care
Open UP 224pp 1996
0-335-19610-1 Hardback £60.00
0-335-19609-8 Paperback £18.99

Malin, N.
Community care for nurses and the caring professions
Open UP 216pp 1999
0-335-19671-3 Hardback £50.00
0-335-19670-5 Paperback £16.99

Malin, N.
Services for people with learning disabilities
Routledge 312pp 2e. Paperback 1994
0-415-09938-2 £16.99

Mandelstam, M.
An A-Z of community care law
Jessica Kingsley 128pp Paperback 1998
1-85302-560-7 £12.95

Mandelstam, M.
Community care practice and the law
Jessica Kingsley 656pp 2e. Paperback 1999
1-85302-647-6 £27.50

Mayer, P.P.
Quality care for elderly people
Arnold 312pp 1997
0-412-61830-3   £55.00

McDonald, A.
Understanding community care
Macmillan Press 288pp Paperback 1999
0-333-67592-4   £13.99

Means, R.
Community care: policy and practice
Macmillan Press 301pp 2e. 1998
0-333-73194-8 Hardback   £47.50
0-333-73195-6 Paperback   £15.50

Ovretveit, J.
Co-ordinating community care
Open UP 240pp Paperback 1993
0-335-19047-2   £19.99

Perkins, R.
Dilemmas in community mental health practice
Radcliffe Medical 160pp Paperback 1998
1-85775-181-7   £19.95

Ritter, S.
Collaborative community mental health care
Arnold 384pp Paperback 1996
0-340-54241-1   £15.99

Sharkey, P.
The essentials of community care
Macmillan Press 192pp Paperback 2000
0-333-77289-X   £13.99

Symonds, A.
The social construction of community care
Macmillan Press 336pp Paperback 1998
0-333-66298-9   £15.99

Victor, C.
Community care and older people
Stanley Thornes 199pp Paperback 1997
0-7487-3292-6   £16.50

Wilmot, S.
The ethics of community care
Continuum Paperback 1996
0-304-33890-7   £14.99

COMPLEMENTARY MEDICINE

Birch, S.
Understanding acupuncture
Churchill Livingstone 340pp 2e. Paperback 1999
0-443-06179-3   £25.00

Brennan, R.
Alexander technique: a practical introduction
Element Books 160pp Paperback 1998
1-86204-158-X   £8.99

Byfield, D.
Chiropractic manipulative skills
Butterworth-Heinemann 224pp Paperback 1995
0-7506-0968-0   £40.00

Dannheisser, L.
An illustrated guide: homeopathy
Element Books 144pp Paperback 1998
1-86204-168-7   £12.99

Downey, P.
Homoeopathy for the primary healthcare team
Butterworth-Heinemann 190pp Paperback 1997
0-7506-2999-1   £17.99

Ernst, E.
Acupuncture: a scientific appraisal
Butterworth-Heinemann 256pp Paperback 1999
0-7506-4163-0   £19.99

Ernst, E.
Complementary medicine: an objective appraisal
Butterworth-Heinemann 176pp Paperback 1996
0-7506-3141-4   £18.99

Ernst, E.
Herbal medicine: a concise overview for professionals
Butterworth-Heinemann 192pp Paperback 1999
0-7506-4540-7   £15.99

Ernst, E.
Homoeopathy: a critical appraisal
Butterworth-Heinemann 192pp Paperback 1998
0-7506-3564-9   £25.00

Fulder, S.
Handbook of alternative and complementary medicine
Oxford UP 340pp 3e. Hardback 1996
0-19-262669-8   £26.50

Hartman, L.
Handbook of osteopathic technique
Stanley Thornes 280pp 3e. Paperback 1996
0-7487-3722-7   £36.50

Jamil, T.
Complementary medicine
Butterworth-Heinemann 267pp Paperback 1997
0-7506-2881-2   £19.99

Newall, C.A.
Herbal medicines
Pharmaceutical Press 312pp Hardback 1996
0-85369-289-0   £35.00

Price, S.
Aromatherapy for health professionals
Churchill Livingstone 394pp 2e. Paperback 1999
0-443-06210-2   £19.50

Rowlands, B.
Which? guide to complementary medicine
Which? Books 272pp Paperback 1997
0-85202-634-X £9.99

Stone, J.
Complementary medicine and the law
Oxford UP 328pp Paperback 1996
0-19-825971-9 £14.99

Vincent, C.
**Complementary medicine: a research
perspective**
John Wiley 312pp Paperback 1997
0-471-96645-2 £27.50

Zollman, C.
ABC of complementary medicine
BMJ Books 56pp 2000
0-7279-1237-2 £16.95

COMPUTING & THE INTERNET

Coiera, E.
**Guide to medical informatics, the Internet and
telemedia**
Arnold 416pp Paperback 1997
0-412-75710-9 £29.99

Dombal, F.T.D.
Medical informatics
Butterworth-Heinemann 133pp Paperback 1996
0-7506-2162-1 £15.99

Gillies, A.
Information and IT for primary care
Radcliffe Medical 136pp Paperback 1999
1-85775-368-2 £21.95

Kiley, R.
The doctor's Internet handbook
Royal Society of Medicine Updated ed Paperback 1998
1-85315-370-2 £8.50

Kiley, R.
Medical information on the Internet
Churchill Livingstone 200pp 2e. Paperback with
CD-ROM 1999
0-443-06194-7 £18.95

Lee, N.
ABC of medical computing
BMJ Books 85pp Paperback 1996
0-7279-1046-9 £17.95

McKenzie, B.C.
Medicine and the Internet
Oxford UP 372pp 2e. Paperback 1997
0-19-262852-6 £17.95

Pallen, M.
Guide to the Internet
BMJ Books 15pp 2e. Paperback 1997
0-7279-1255-0 £5.95

Tyrrell, S.
Using the Internet in healthcare
Radcliffe Medical 168pp Paperback 1999
1-85775-366-6 £17.95

Yates, F.E.
Creative computing in health and social care
John Wiley 236pp Paperback 1996
0-471-95586-8 £45.00

COUNSELLING

Bayne, R.
**Counselling and communication skills for
medical and health practitioners**
British Psychological Society 176pp Paperback 1998
1-85433-256-2 £14.50

Bayne, R.
Counsellors' handbook
Stanley Thornes 207pp Paperback 1999
0-7487-3309-4 £19.00

Burnard, P.
Counselling skills for health professionals
Stanley Thornes 272pp 3e. Paperback 1999
0-7487-3976-9 £20.00

Davies, D.
Counselling in psychological services
Open UP 160pp Paperback 1997
0-335-19164-9 £15.99

Dryden, W.
Handbook of individual therapy
Sage London 432pp Hardback 1996
0-8039-7843-X Paperback £18.99
0-8039-7842-1 Hardback £49.50

East, P.
Counselling in medical settings
Open UP 163pp Paperback 1995
0-335-19241-6 £15.99

Egan, G.
The skilled helper
Brooks Cole 388pp 6e. Hardback 1998
0-534-34948-X £22.99

Feltham, C.
Understanding the counselling relationship
Sage London 304pp 1999
0-7619-5784-7 Hardback £45.00
0-7619-5785-5 Paperback £14.99

Keithley, J.
Counselling in primary health care
Oxford UP 324pp Hardback 1995
0-19-262354-0 £32.50

McLeod, J.
An introduction to counselling
Open UP 457pp 2e. Paperback 1998
0-335-19709-4 £17.99

Mearns, D.
Person-centred counselling in action
Sage London 176pp 2e. 1999
0-7619-6316-2 Hardback £40.00
0-7619-6317-0 Paperback £12.99

Nelson-Jones, R.
Introduction to counselling skills
Sage London 256pp 1999
0-7619-6185-2 Hardback £49.50
0-7619-6186-0 Paperback £18.99

Nelson-Jones, R.
The theory and practice of counselling
Continuum 360pp 2e. Paperback 1995
0-304-33137-6 £19.99

Palmer, S.
Counselling in a multicultural society
Sage London 224pp 1998
0-7619-5064-8 Hardback £37.50
0-7619-5065-6 Paperback £13.99

Payne, R.A.
Relaxation techniques
Churchill Livingstone 224pp Paperback 1995
0-443-04933-5 £23.95

Scrutton, S.
Counselling older people
Arnold 247pp 2e. Paperback 1999
0-340-71948-6 £13.99

Tschudin, V.
Counselling for loss and bereavement
Bailliere Tindall 168pp 1997
0-7020-2131-8 £12.95

Wiener, J.
Counselling and psychotherapy in primary health care
Macmillan Press 192pp Paperback 1998
0-333-65205-3 £12.99

DENTISTRY & ORAL MEDICINE

Andlaw, R.J.
A manual of paediatric dentistry
Churchill Livingstone 249pp 4e. Paperback 1996
0-443-05372-3 £31.00

Cawson, R.A.
Essentials of oral pathology and oral medicine
Churchill Livingstone 384pp 6e. Paperback 1998
0-443-05348-0 £36.00

Cawson, R.A.
Lucas's pathology of tumors of the oral tissues
Churchill Livingstone 400pp 5e. Hardback 1998
0-443-03990-9 £122.00

Eveson, J.
Color atlas of oral pathology
Mosby 128pp Hardback 1995
0-7234-2112-9 £39.95

Fairpo, J.E.H.
Heinemann dental dictionary
Wright 352pp 4e. Paperback 1997
0-7506-2208-3 £17.99

Harty, F.J.
Harty's endodontics in clinical practice
Wright 288pp 4e. Paperback 1997
0-7236-1020-7 £30.00

Jones, M.L.
Walther & Houston's orthodontic notes
Wright 288pp 6e. Paperback 2000
0-7236-1065-7 £19.50

Kidd, E.A.M.
Pickard's manual of operative dentistry
Oxford UP 208pp 7e. Paperback 1996
0-19-262609-4 £29.95

Lamey, P.
A clinical guide to oral medicine
Macmillan Journals 96pp 2e. Paperback 1997
0-904588-50-5 £26.95

Manson, J.D.
Outline of periodontics
Wright 320pp 4e. Paperback 1999
0-7236-1070-3 £29.99

Marsh, P.D.
Oral microbiology
Wright 224pp 4e. Paperback 1999
0-7236-1051-7 £27.50

Mason, R.
A guide to dental radiography
Oxford UP 272pp 4e. Paperback 1998
0-19-262672-8 Hardback £65.00
0-19-262671-X Paperback £32.50

McCabe, J.F.
Applied dental materials
Blackwell Science UK 256pp 8e. Paperback 1998
0-632-04208-7 £27.50

McGowan, D.
Atlas of minor oral surgery
Martin Dunitz 22. 1999
1-85317-766-0 £39.95

Mitchell, L.
Oxford handbook of clinical dentistry
Oxford UP 818pp 3e. Plastic-reinforced paper 1999
0-19-262963-8 £17.95

Pine, C.
Community oral health
Wright 336pp Paperback 1996
0-7236-1095-9 £27.50

Scully, C.
Handbook of oral disease
Martin Dunitz 300pp Hardback 1999
1-85317-615-X £45.00

Scully, C.
Medical problems in dentistry
Wright 400pp 4e. Hardback 1998
0-7236-1056-8 £45.00

Scully, C.
Oxford handbook of dental patient care
Oxford UP 456pp Paperback 1998
0-19-262915-8 £18.95

Smith, B.G.N.
Planning and making crowns and bridges
Martin Dunitz 264pp 3e. Hardback 1998
1-85317-314-2 £49.95

Soames, J.V.
Oral pathology
Oxford UP 352pp 3e. 1998
0-19-262895-X Hardback £75.00
0-19-262894-1 Paperback £29.95

Tyldesley, W.R.
Oral medicine
Oxford UP 180pp 4e. 1995
0-19-262626-4 Hardback £55.00
0-19-262625-6 Paperback £29.95

Whaites, E.
Essentials of dental radiography and radiology
Churchill Livingstone 416pp 2e. Paperback 1996
0-443-05349-9 £39.00

DERMATOLOGY

Baran, R.
A text atlas of nail disorders
Martin Dunitz 288pp 2e. Hardback 1996
1-85317-201-4 £49.95

Berker, D.
Handbook of diseases of the nails and their management
Blackwell Science USA 184pp Paperback 1995
0-86542-907-3 £39.50

Buxton, P.K.
ABC of dermatology
BMJ Books 120pp 3e. Paperback 1998
0-7279-1150-3 £17.95

Champion, R.H.
Textbook of dermatology
Blackwell Science UK 3840pp 6e. 4 vols 1998
0-632-03796-2 Hardback £395.00
0-632-04904-9 CD-ROM £346.63

Cox, N.H.
Diagnostic problems in dermatology
Mosby 192pp Hardback 1998
0-7234-2790-9 £28.95

Dawber, R.
Cutaneous cryosurgery
Martin Dunitz 200pp 2e. Hardback 1997
1-85317-430-0 £49.95

Dawber, R.
Diseases of the hair and scalp
Blackwell Science UK 616pp 3e. Hardback 1997
0-86542-866-2 £125.00

Eedy, D.J.
Surgical dermatology
Blackwell Science UK 272pp Hardback 1996
0-632-03425-4 £49.50

Elder, D.E.
Lever's histopathology of the skin
Williams and Wilkins 1104pp 8e. Hardback 1997
0-397-51500-6 £129.00

Fitzpatrick, T.B.
Color atlas and synopsis of clinical dermatology
McGraw-Hill USA 1030pp 3e. 1997
0-07-021388-7 Paperback £39.99
0-07-913204-9 With CD-ROM £93.99

Freedberg, I.M.
Fitzpatrick's dermatology in general medicine
McGraw-Hill USA 3120pp 5e. 2 vols Hardback 1999
0-07-912938-2 £270.00

Fry, L.
An atlas of practical dermatology
Parthenon 212pp Hardback 1997
1-85070-461-9 £68.00

Gawkrodger, D.
Dermatology
Churchill Livingstone 136pp 2e. Paperback 1997
0-443-05328-6 £21.95

Graham-Brown, R.
Color atlas and text of dermatology
Mosby 320pp Paperback 1998
0-7234-2421-7 £26.95

Graham-Brown, R.A.C.
Lecture notes on dermatology
Blackwell Science UK 288pp 7e. Paperback 1996
0-86542-635-X   £14.95

Gray, J.
A pocket book of hair and scalp disorders
Blackwell Science UK 112pp Paperback 1998
0-632-05189-2   £14.95

Hunter, J.A.A.
Clinical dermatology
Blackwell Science UK 328pp 2e. Paperback 1995
0-632-03714-8   £21.50

Mackie, R.M.
Clinical dermatology
Oxford UP 340pp 4e. 1997
0-19-262763-5 Hardback   £45.00
0-19-262761-9 Paperback   £19.95

MacKie, R.M.
Skin cancer
Martin Dunitz 368pp 2e. Hardback 1996
1-85317-203-0   £75.00

Marks, R.
Practical problems in dermatology
Martin Dunitz 264pp 2e. Paperback 1996
1-85317-050-X   £25.00

Marks, R.
Skin disease in old age
Martin Dunitz 288pp 2e. Hardback 1998
1-85317-227-8   £49.95

McKee, P.H.
Essential skin pathology
Mosby 256pp Paperback 1999
0-7234-3067-5   £39.95

McKee, P.H.
Pathology of the skin
Mosby 848pp 2e. Hardback 1996
1-56375-588-2   £245.00

Rycroft, R.J.G.
A colour handbook of dermatology
Manson Publishing 288pp 1999
1-874545-25-1   £29.95

Savin, A.
Color atlas of skin signs in clinical medicine
Mosby 256pp Paperback 1996
0-7234-2240-0   £25.95

White, G.
Levene's color atlas of dermatology
Mosby 384pp 2e. Paperback 1996
0-7234-2552-3   £21.95

Wilkinson, J.D.
Dermatology
Churchill Livingstone 160pp 2e. 1998
0-443-05852-0   £11.95

DIAGNOSIS & CLINICAL METHODS
(See also Medicine, Surgery)

Beck, E.R.
Tutorials in differential diagnosis
Churchill Livingstone 272pp 4e. Paperback 2001
0-443-06157-2   £17.50

Bouchier, I.A.D.
French's index of differential diagnosis
Butterworth-Heinemann 827pp 13e. Hardback 1996
0-7506-1434-X   £45.00

Epstein, O.
Clinical examination
Mosby 432pp 2e. 1997
0-7234-2576-0 Paperback   £31.95
0-7234-2184-6 CD-ROM   £82.19

Ford, M.J.
Introduction to clinical examination
Churchill Livingstone 152pp 7e. Paperback 2000
0-443-06354-0   £11.95

Mir, A.
Atlas of clinical diagnosis
W B Saunders Co 276pp Paperback 1995
0-7020-1846-5   £25.95

Mir, M.A.
Atlas of clinical skills
W B Saunders 320pp Paperback 1997
0-7020-1816-3   £21.95

Munro, J.F.
MacLeod's clinical examination
Churchill Livingstone 324pp 10e. Paperback 2000
0-443-06172-6   £21.95

Ogilvie, C.
Chamberlain's symptoms and signs in clinical medicine
Butterworth-Heinemann 448pp 12e. Paperback 1997
0-7506-2030-7   £35.00

Pounder, R.E.
Handbook of current diagnosis and treatment
Churchill Livingstone 494pp Paperback 1996
0-443-05600-5   £23.00

Scott, N.A.
Procedures in practice
BMJ Books 288pp 3e. Paperback 1994
0-7279-0823-5   £15.95

Swash, M.
Hutchison's clinical methods
W B Saunders Co 512pp 20e. Paperback 1995
0-7020-1675-6   £16.95

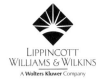

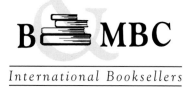

Talley, N.J.
Clinical examination: a guide to physical diagnosis
Blackwell Science 500pp 3e. Paperback 1996
0-86542-689-9 £17.95

Talley, N.J.
Pocket clinical examination
Blackwell Science UK 204pp Paperback 1998
0-632-05152-3 £12.95

Toghill, P.J.
Essential medical procedures
Arnold 160pp Paperback 1996
0-340-63187-2 £19.99

Turner, R.C.
Lecture notes on clinical skills
Blackwell Science UK 336pp 3e. Paperback 1997
0-86542-971-5 £12.95

Welsby, P.D.
Clinical history taking and examination
Churchill Livingstone 172pp Paperback 1996
0-443-04328-0 £19.95

DICTIONARIES & REFERENCE
(See also Health Administration)

Concise medical dictionary
Oxford UP 726pp 5e. 1998
0-19-262916-6 Hardback £18.99
0-19-280075-2 Paperback £8.99

Dorlands illustrated medical dictionary
W B Saunders 1974pp 29e. Hardback 2000
0-7216-6254-4 £31.95

International statistical classification of diseases and related health problems (ICD-10)
WHO 1248pp 3 vols 10th revision Hardback 1992
92-4-154419-8 (Vol. 1: Tabular List) £75.00
92-4-154420-1 (Vol. 2: Instruction manual) £25.00
92-4-154421-X (Vol. 3: Alphabetical index) £85.00

Anderson, K.N.
Mosby's medical, nursing, and allied health dictionary
Mosby 2112pp 5e. Hardback 1998
1-55664-566-X £22.95

Chapman, M.D.
Charities digest 2000
Waterlow Professional Publications Paperback 1999
1-85783-859-9 £21.95

Corps, L.
The insider's guide to medical schools
BMJ Books 170pp 2e. Paperback 1999
0-7279-1428-6 £14.95

Crombie, I.K.
The pocket guide to grant applications
BMJ Books 68pp Mixed-media pack 1998
0-7279-1219-4 £16.95

Dale, P.
Guide to libraries and information sources in medicine and health care
British Library 187pp 2e. Paperback 1997
0-7123-0839-3 £39.00

Davis, J.
The directory of grant-making trusts 1999-2000
Charities Aid Foundation 3 vols Paperback 1999
1-85934-078-4 £89.95

Firkin, B.G.
Dictionary of medical eponyms
Parthenon 590pp 2e. Hardback 1996
1-85070-477-5 £35.00

Forrester, W.H.
Directory of medical and health care libraries in the United Kingdom and Republic of Ireland 2000-2001
Library Association 288pp 11e. Paperback 2000
1-85604-378-9 £35.00

Gatrell, J.
The specialist registrar handbook
Radcliffe Medical 320pp Paperback 1999
1-85775-361-5 £21.50

Grantfinder - medicine
Macmillan Reference 392pp Hardback 1999
0-333-77729-8 £24.99

Jablonski, S.
Dictionary of medical acronyms and abbreviations
Hanley Belfus 450pp 3e. Paperback 1998
1-56053-264-5 £13.95

Jablonski, S.
Jablonski's dictionary of syndromes and eponymic diseases
Krieger Publishing 680pp 2e. Hardback 1991
0-89464-224-3 £93.95

Johnson, C.J.H.
Getting ahead in medicine
Bios Scientific 192pp Paperback 1998
1-85996-021-9 £17.95

Keighley, B.
Guide to postgraduate medical education
BMJ Books 184pp Paperback 1996
0-7279-1072-8 £18.95

Lock, S.
The Oxford illustrated companion to medicine
Oxford UP 1008pp 3e. Hardback 2000
0-19-262950-6 £39.50

MacPherson, G.
Black's medical dictionary
A & C Black 636pp Hardback 1999
0-7136-4566-0   £25.00

Macpherson, G.
Our NHS: a celebration of 50 years
BMJ Books 242pp Hardback 1998
0-7279-1279-8   £25.00

Magalini, S.I.
Dictionary of medical syndromes
Williams and Wilkins 976pp 4e. Hardback 1997
0-397-58418-0   £76.00

Medical directory 2000
Informa Publishing Group 2 vols 2000
1-85978-554-9   £178.00

Medical register 2000
General Medical Council 4 vols 2000
No ISBN   £110.00

Morton, L.
A bibliography of medical and biomedical biography
Scolar Press 350pp 2e. Hardback 1994
0-85967-981-0   £75.00

Norman, J.M.
Morton's medical bibliography
Scolar Press 1272pp 5e. Hardback 1991
0-85967-897-0   £131.50

Parkinson, J.
Manual of English for the overseas doctor
Churchill Livingstone 296pp 5e. Paperback 1998
0-443-06136-X   £18.95

Porter, R.
The Cambridge illustrated history of medicine
Cambridge UP 400pp Hardback 1996
0-521-44211-7   £24.95

Quarini, C.A.
Medical training and working in the UK
PasTest 96pp 3e. Paperback 1997
0-906896-97-5   £12.95

Reece, D.
How to do it
BMJ Books 3 vols 3e. Paperback 1995
0-7279-0906-1   £38.00

Richards, P.
Learning medicine
BMJ Books 128pp 15e. Paperback 2000
0-7279-1462-6   £14.95

Smith, T.
The BMA complete family health encyclopedia
Dorling Kindersley 3e. Hardback 2000
0-7513-0795-5   £35.00

Stedmans medical dictionary
Williams and Wilkins 2336pp 27e. Hardback 2000
0-683-40007-X   £29.95

The voluntary agencies directory
NCVO Publications 516pp 19e. Paperback 2000
0-7199-1552-X   £22.50

World directory of medical schools
WHO 338pp 7e. Paperback 2000
9-24-150010-7   £25.00

Wingate, P.
The Penguin medical encyclopedia
Penguin 688pp 4e. Paperback 1996
0-14-051361-2   £9.99

EAR, NOSE & THROAT
(See also Speech & Language Therapy)

Ballenger, J.J.
Otorhinolaryngology
Williams and Wilkins 1404pp 15e. Hardback 1996
0-683-00315-1   £125.00

Bleach, N.
Operative otorhinolaryngology
Blackwell Science UK 512pp Hardback 1997
0-632-03747-4   £175.00

Browning, G.G.
Clinical otology and audiology
Butterworth-Heinemann 320pp 2e. Paperback 1998
0-7506-3373-5   £45.00

Bull, P.D.
Lecture notes on diseases of the ear, nose and throat
Blackwell Science USA 208pp 8e. Paperback 1996
0-86542-634-1   £14.95

Bull, T.R.
A colour atlas of ENT diagnosis
Mosby 3e. Paperback 1995
0-7234-2271-0   £21.95

Burton, M.J.
Hall and Colman's diseases of the ear, nose and throat
Churchill Livingstone 244pp 15e. Paperback 2000
0-443-06190-4   £21.95

Corbridge, R.
Modern ENT practice
Arnold 192pp Paperback 1998
0-340-67704-X   £17.99

Dhillon, R.S.
Ear, nose and throat and head and neck surgery
Churchill Livingstone 136pp 2e. Paperback 1999
0-443-05955-1   £20.00

Drake-Lee, A.
Clinical otorhinolaryngology
Churchill Livingstone 267pp Paperback 1995
0-443-04965-3 £17.95

Hawke, M.
Diagnostic handbook of otorhinolaryngology
Martin Dunitz 304pp Hardback 1997
1-85317-383-5 £19.95

Hawthorne, M.R.
Synopsis of otolaryngology
Butterworth-Heinemann 6e. 2000
0-7506-4240-8 £55.00

Kerr, A.G.
Scott-Brown's otolaryngology
Butterworth-Heinemann 3928pp 6 vols 6e.
Hardback 1997
0-7506-1935-X £700.00

Ludman, H.
ABC of otolaryngology
BMJ Books 72pp 4e. Paperback 1997
0-7279-1205-4 £16.95

Ludman, H.
Diseases of the ear
Arnold 588pp 6e. Hardback 1997
0-340-56441-5 £100.00

Maran, A.G.D.
Logan Turner's diseases of the ear, nose and throat
Butterworth-Heinemann 11e. Paperback 2000
0-7506-2399-3 £25.00

Milford, C.
Shared care for ENT
Isis Medical Media 194pp 1999
1-899066-69-1 £22.50

Wilson, J.A.
Stell & Maran's head and neck surgery
Butterworth-Heinemann 384pp 4e. Hardback 2000
0-7506-3366-2 £85.00

ENDOCRINOLOGY & DIABETES

Alberti, K.G.M.M.
International textbook of diabetes mellitus
John Wiley 1930pp 2e. Hardback 1997
0-471-93930-7 £225.00

Besser, G.M.
Clinical endocrinology
Mosby 432pp 2e. Hardback 1994
1-56375-552-1 £129.00

Brook, C.G.D.
Essential endocrinology
Blackwell Science UK 192pp 3e. Paperback 1996
0-632-03622-2 £17.95

Clarke, J.T.R.
A clinical guide to inherited metabolic diseases
Cambridge UP 300pp 1996
0-521-48064-7 Hardback £60.00
0-521-48524-X Paperback £24.95

Fox, C.
Diabetes in the real world
Class Publishing 288pp 1995
1-872362-53-2 £19.95

Gatling, W.
Shared care for diabetes
Isis Medical Media 200pp 1997
1-899066-25-X £22.50

Grossman, A.
Clinical endocrinology
Blackwell Science 1200pp 2e. 1997
0-86542-629-5 £235.00

Hadley, M.E.
Endocrinology
Prentice Hall 585pp 5e. Paperback 1999
0-13-080356-1 £42.99

Jones, E.
An illustrated guide for the diabetic clinic
Blackwell Science UK 152pp Paperback 1998
0-632-05151-5 £16.95

Laycock, J.F.
Essential endocrinology
Oxford UP 3e. 1996
0-19-262472-5 Hardback £47.50
0-19-262471-7 Paperback £19.95

Levy, A.
Endocrinology
Oxford UP 410pp Paperback 1997
0-19-262766-X £17.95

Page, S.R.
Diabetes: emergency and hospital management
BMJ Books 248pp Paperback 1999
0-7279-1229-1 £25.00

Pickup, J.C.
Textbook of diabetes
Blackwell Science UK 1600pp 2 vols 2e.
Hardback 1996
0-632-03802-0 £195.00

Scriver, C.R.
The metabolic basis of inherited disease
3 vols McGraw-Hill HPD 3008pp 7e.1995
0-07-909826-6 Hardback £240.00
0-07-864187-X (CD-ROM 1997) £299.99

Watkins, P.
ABC of diabetes
BMJ Books 75pp 4e. Paperback 1998
0-7279-1189-9 £14.95

Watkins, P.J.
Diabetes and its management
Blackwell Science UK 320pp 5e. Paperback 1996
0-86542-863-8 £24.95

Williams, G.
Handbook of diabetes
Blackwell Science UK 224pp 2e. Paperback 1999
0-632-05504-9 £29.95

Wilson, J.D.
Williams textbook of endocrinology
W B Saunders 1632pp 9e. Hardback 1998
0-7216-6152-1 £115.00

EPIDEMIOLOGY & STATISTICS
(See also Public Health & Social Medicine)

Altman, D.
Statistics with confidence
BMJ Books 200pp 2e. Hardback 2000
0-7279-1375-1 £15.95

Armitage, P.
Statistical methods in medical research
Blackwell Science UK 640pp 3e. Hardback 1994
0-632-03695-8 £42.50

Barker, D.J.P.
Epidemiology in medical practice
Churchill Livingstone 178pp Paperback 5e. 1998
0-443-05620-X £13.95

Beaglehole, R.
Basic epidemiology
WHO 171pp 1993
92-4-154446-5 £11.25

Bland, M.
An introduction to medical statistics
Oxford UP 410pp 2e. Paperback 1995
0-19-262428-8 £18.95

Campbell, M.
Statistics at square one
BMJ Books 146pp 9e. Paperback 1996
0-7279-0916-9 £9.95

Campbell, M.J.
Medical statistics: a commonsense approach
John Wiley 218pp 3e. Paperback 1999
0-471-98721-2 £16.99

Coggon, D.
Epidemiology for the uninitiated
BMJ Books 69pp 4e. 1997
0-7279-1102-3 £10.95

Coggon, D.
Statistics in clinical practice
BMJ Books 120pp 1995
0-7279-0907-X £11.95

Compendium of health statistics
Office of Health Economics 12e. 2000
Book (Public sector) £70.00
Book and CD-ROM (Public sector) £152.25

Daly, L.
Interpretation and uses of medical statistics
Blackwell Science UK 576pp 5e. Paperback 2000
0-632-04763-1 £35.00

Fletcher, R.H.
Clinical epidemiology
Williams and Wilkins 304pp 3e. Paperback 1996
0-683-03269-0 £19.95

Friedman, G.D.
Primer of epidemiology
McGraw-Hill HPD 336pp 4e. Paperback 1994
0-07-022454-4 £21.99

Gordis, L.
Epidemiology
W B Saunders 320pp 2e. Paperback 2000
0-7216-8338-X £19.95

Health and personal social services statistics for England
Stationery Office Paperback 1999
0-11-322306-4 £17.50

Last, J.M.
A dictionary of epidemiology
Oxford UP Inc 198pp 3e. Paperback 1995
0-19-509668-1 £17.95

MacMahon, B.
Epidemiology: principles and methods
Little, Brown 360pp 2e. 1996
0-316-54222-9 £29.50

Matthews, J.
Introduction to randomised controlled clinical trials
Arnold 208pp Paperback 2000
0-340-76143-1 £19.99

Petrie, A.
Medical statistics at a glance
Blackwell Science 136pp Paperback 2000
0-632-05075-6 £12.95

Sackett, D.
Clinical epidemiology: a basic science for clinical medicine
Williams and Wilkins 441pp 2e. Paperback 1991
0-316-76599-6 £30.00

Vetter, N.J.
Epidemiology and public health medicine
Churchill Livingstone 272pp Paperback 1999
0-443-05704-4   £15.95

EVIDENCE-BASED MEDICINE

Chalmers, I.
Systematic reviews
BMJ Books 128pp Paperback 1995
0-7279-0904-5   £15.95

Chambers, R.
Clinical effectiveness made easy
Radcliffe Medical 136pp Paperback 1998
1-85775-316-X   £17.95

Cochrane, A.
Effectiveness and efficiency
Royal Society Medicine Paperback 1999
1-85315-394-X   £8.95

Crombie, I.K.
The pocket guide to critical appraisal
BMJ Books 80pp Paperback 1996
0-7279-1099-X   £10.95

Dixon, R.A.
Evidence-based medicine
Butterworth-Heinemann 160pp Paperback 1997
0-7506-2590-2   £17.99

Dunning, M.
Turning evidence into everyday practice
King's Fund 80pp Paperback 1997
1-85717-151-9   £9.99

Evans, D.
Implementing evidence-based changes in healthcare
Radcliffe Medical 344pp Paperback 2000
1-85775-382-8   £27.50

Gray, M.
Evidence based health care
Churchill Livingstone 300pp 2e. Paperback 2000
0-443-06288-9   £22.50

Greenhalgh, T.
Evidence based health care workbook
BMJ Books 128pp Paperback 1999
0-7279-1447-2   £19.95

Greenhalgh, T.
How to read a paper
BMJ Books 184pp Paperback 1997
0-7279-1139-2   £14.95

Haines, A.
Getting research findings into practice
BMJ Books 170pp Paperback 1998
0-7279-1257-7   £19.95

Jadad, A.R.
Randomised controlled trials
BMJ Books 138pp Paperback 1998
0-7279-1208-9   £12.95

Lancaster, T.
Practising evidence-based primary care
Radcliffe Medical 163pp Paperback 1999
1-85775-405-0   £30.00

Lockett, T.
Evidence-based and cost-effective medicine for the uninitiated
Radcliffe Medical 104pp Paperback 1997
1-85775-235-X   £16.95

Lugon, M.
Clinical governance: making it happen
Royal Society of Medicine 232pp Paperback 1999
1-85315-383-4   £17.50

Maynard, A.
Non-random reflections on health service resources
BMJ Books 109pp Paperback 1997
0-7279-1151-1   £25.00

Miles, A.
Effective clinical practice
Blackwell Science UK 264pp Paperback 1996
0-632-03908-6   £18.99

Po, A.L.W.
Dictionary of evidence-based medicine
Radcliffe Medical 120pp Paperback 1998
1-85775-305-4   £19.95

Ridsdale, L.
Evidence based practice in primary care
Churchill Livingstone 176pp Paperback 1998
0-443-05889-X   £17.95

Sackett, D.
Evidence-based medicine: how to practice and teach EBM
Churchill Livingston 275pp 2e. Hardback with CD-ROM 2000
0-443-06240-4   £18.95

Silagy, C.
Evidence based practice in primary care
BMJ Books 198pp Paperback 1998
0-7279-1210-0   £25.00

FORENSIC MEDICINE & MEDICAL LAW
(See also Legislation, Medical Ethics)

Action for Victims of Medical Accidents: Medical accidents and the law
Wiley Law 448pp 1998
0-471-96642-8   £24.95

British Medical Association
Assessment of mental capacity: guidance for doctors and lawyers
BMA Professional 52pp Paperback 1995
0-7279-0913-4 £8.95

Davies, M.
Textbook on medical law
Blackstone Press 431pp 2e. Paperback 1998
1-85431-842-X £21.95

Dorries, C.
Coroners courts
John Wiley 432pp Hardback 1999
0-471-96721-1 £34.95

Finch, J.
Speller's law relating to hospitals
Arnold 968pp 7e. Hardback 1993
0-412-41000-1 £140.00

Gunn, J.
Forensic psychiatry
Butterworth-Heinemann 1100pp 2e. Hardback 2001
0-7506-4183-5 £150.00

Healy, J.
Medical negligence
Sweet & Maxwell 200pp 1999
0-421-68060-1 £23.95

Hurwitz, B.
Clinical guidelines and the law
Radcliffe Medical 152pp Paperback 1998
1-85775-044-6 £19.95

Jones, M.A.
Blackstone's statutes on medical law
Blackstone Press 446pp 2e. Paperback 1999
1-85431-709-1 £16.95

Kennedy, I.
Principles of medical law
Oxford UP 1076pp Hardback 1999
0-19-829888-9 £145.00

Khan, M.
Medical negligence
Cavendish 462pp Paperback 1997
1-85941-022-7 £34.95

Knight, B.
Forensic pathology
Arnold 648pp 2e. Hardback 1996
0-340-58897-7 £150.00

Knight, B.
Simpson's forensic medicine
Arnold 224pp 11e. Paperback 1997
0-340-61370-X £32.50

Leung, W-C.
Law for doctors
Blackwell Science UK 224pp Paperback 2000
0-632-05243-0 £24.95

Lewis, C.
Medical negligence: a practical guide
Butterworths 627pp 4e. Hardback 1998
0-406-90283-6 £60.00

Marquand, P.B.
An introduction to medical law
Butterworth-Heinemann 136pp Paperback 2000
0-7506-4239-4 £15.99

Mason, K.
The pathology of trauma
Arnold 624pp 3e. Hardback 1999
0-340-69189-1 £155.00

McHale, J.
Health care law: text, cases and materials
Sweet & Maxwell 974pp Paperback 1997
0-421-51180-X £29.95

Montague, A.
Legal problems in emergency medicine
Oxford UP 176pp 1996
0-19-262497-0 Hardback £29.95
0-19-262496-2 Paperback £16.95

Montgomery, J.
Health care law
Oxford UP 532pp 1997
0-19-876260-7 Hardback £50.00
0-19-876259-3 Paperback £20.99

Phillips, A.F.
Medical negligence law: seeking a balance
Dartmouth 248pp 1997
1-85521-643-4 £47.00

Powers, M.
Clinical negligence
Butterworths Law 3e. Hardback
0-406-92461-9 £295.00

Stauch, M.
Sourcebook on medical law
Cavendish Publishing 758pp Paperback 1998
1-85941-103-7 £27.95

Stone, J.H.
Faulk's basic forensic psychiatry
Blackwell Science UK 352pp 3e. Paperback 1999
0-632-05019-5 £26.50

Williams, D.J.
Forensic pathology
Churchill Livingstone 139pp Paperback 1997
0-443-05388-X £11.95

GASTROENTEROLOGY

Bircher, J.
Oxford textbook of clinical hepatology
2 vols Oxford UP 1792pp 2e.Hardback 1999
0-19-262515-2 £275.00

Cope, Z.
Cope's early diagnosis of the acute abdomen
Oxford UP Inc 320pp 20e Paperback 2000
0-19-513679-9 £22.50

Cotton, P.B.
Practical gastrointestinal endoscopy
Blackwell Science USA 352pp 4e. Hardback 1996
0-86542-851-4 £52.50

Dalton, H.R.
Key topics in gastroenterology
Bios Scientific 250pp Paperback 1998
1-85996-281-5 £21.95

Farthing, M.J.G.
Drug therapy for gastrointestinal disease
Martin Dunitz 300pp Hardback 2001
1-85317-733-4 £49.95

Feldman, M.
**Sleisenger & Fordtran's gastrointestinal and liver
disease**
W B Saunders 2336pp 6e. Hardback 1997
0-7216-6291-9 £146.00

Garden, O.J.
Hepatobiliary and pancreatic surgery
W B Saunders 320pp Hardback 1997
0-7020-2142-3 £49.95

Griffin, S.M.
Upper-gastrointestinal surgery
W B Saunders 448pp Hardback 1997
0-7020-2141-5 £49.95

Heatley, R.V.
The Helicobacter pylori handbook
Blackwell Science UK 80pp 2e. Paperback 1998
0-632-05176-0 £12.95

Jones, D.J.M.F.
ABC of colorectal diseases
BMJ Books 120pp 2e. Paperback 1998
0-7279-1105-8 £18.95

Kamm, M.A.
Inflammatory bowel disease
Martin Dunitz 72pp Paperback 1999
1-85317-641-9 £9.95

Keighley, M.R.B.
Surgery of the anus, rectum & colon
2 vols W B Saunders 2872pp 2e. Hardback 1999
0-7020-2335-3 £285.00

MacSween, R.N.M.
Pathology of the liver
Churchill Livingstone 816pp 3e. Hardback 1995
0-443-04454-6 £260.00

McDonald, J.
Evidence based gastroenterology and hepatology
BMJ Books 572pp Hardback 1999
0-7279-1182-1 £75.00

Neiman, R.S.
Disorders of the spleen
W B Saunders 320pp Hardback 1999
0-7216-7551-4 £55.00

Nicholls, R.J.
Surgery of the colon and rectum
Churchill Livingstone 1300pp Hardback 1997
0-443-05565-3 £195.00
0-443-05649-8 CD-ROM £205.63

Phillips, R.K.S.
Colorectal surgery
W B Saunders 380pp Hardback 1997
0-7020-2143-1 £49.95

Pounder, R.E.
A colour atlas of the digestive system
Mosby 232pp Paperback 1993
0-7234-1953-1 £30.00

Rhodes, J.M.
Clinical problems in gastroenterology
Mosby 320pp Paperback 1995
0-7234-1943-4 £35.00

Shearman, D.J.C.
Diseases of the gastrointestinal tract and liver
Churchill Livingstone 1518pp 3e. Hardback 1997
0-443-05147-X £209.00

Shepherd, M.
Practical endoscopy
Arnold 464pp 2e. Paperback 1997
0-412-54000-2 £45.00

Sherlock, S.
Diseases of the liver and biliary system
Blackwell Science UK 704pp 10e. Hardback 1996
0-86542-906-5 £69.50

Travis, S.P.L.
Pocket consultant: gastroenterology
Blackwell Science UK 528pp 2e. Paperback 1998
0-632-04887-5 £29.95

Zinner, M.J.
Maingot's abdominal operations
2 vols Appleton and Lange 2176pp 10e.
Hardback 1997
0-8385-6106-3 £179.00

GENERAL PRACTICE

Balint, M.
The doctor, his patient and the illness
Churchill Livingstone 416pp New e Hardback 2000
0-443-06460-1 £35.00

Birch, K.
Quality in general practice
Radcliffe Medical 160pp Paperback 2000
1-85775-364-X   £19.95

Brown, J.S.
Minor surgery
Arnold 480pp 4e. Hardback 2000
0-340-76113-X   £85.00

Brown, J.S.
Procedures in general practice
BMJ Books 192pp Paperback 1997
0-7279-1035-3   £27.00

Carter, Y.
Handbook of sexual health in primary care
Royal Col of General 208pp Paperback 1997
0-85084-238-7   £18.00

Carter, Y.
Research methods in primary care
Radcliffe Medical 200pp Paperback 1996
1-85775-198-1   £19.95

Carter, Y.
Research opportunities in primary care
Radcliffe Medical 256pp Paperback 1999
1-85775-242-2   £18.95

Cartwright, S.
Churchill's pocketbook of general practice
Churchill Livingstone 360pp Paperback 1998
0-443-04863-0   £15.95

Chambers, R.
Survival skills for GPs
Radcliffe Medical 176pp Paperback 1999
1-85775-334-8   £30.00

Chambers, R.
What stress in primary care?
Royal Col of General Practitioners 187pp
Paperback 1999
0-85084-245-X   £19.99

Dean, J.
Making sense of practice finance
Radcliffe Medical 256pp 3e. Paperback 2000
1-85775-331-3   £19.95

Ellis, N.
General practice employment handbook
Radcliffe Medical 180pp Paperback 1998
1-85775-234-1   £17.95

Ellis, N.
General practioners handbook
Radcliffe Medical 216pp 2e. Paperback 2000
1-85775-406-9   £17.95

Elwyn, G.
Integrated teams in primary care
Radcliffe Medical 144pp Paperback 1998
1-85775-288-0   £18.95

Finlay, R.D.
The eye in general practice
Butterworth-Heinemann 212pp 10e. Paperback 1997
0-7506-3691-2   £27.50

Fraser, R.C.
Clinical method: a general practice approach
Butterworth-Heinemann 192pp 3e. Paperback 1999
0-7506-4005-7   £18.99

Freeman, R.
Mentoring in general practice
Butterworth-Heinemann 192pp Paperback 1998
0-7506-3940-7   £22.50

Fry, J.
Common diseases
Petroc Press 440pp 4e. Hardback 1993
0-7923-8803-8   £24.95

Gabbay, M.
Evidence based primary care handbook
RSM Press Paperback 1999
1-85315-415-6   £19.50

Greenhalgh, T.
Quality in general practice
King's Fund 80pp Paperback 1999
1-85717-266-3   £8.99

Hall, M.
GP training handbook
Blackwell Science UK 256pp 3e. Paperback 1999
0-632-05039-X   £24.95

Harrison, J.
GP tomorrow
Radcliffe Medical 216pp Paperback 1998
1-85775-203-1   £18.95

Hobbs, R.
Prescribing in primary care
Oxford UP 228pp Paperback 1998
0-19-262687-6   £19.95

Hopcroft, K.
Symptom sorter
Radcliffe Medical 264pp Paperback 1999
1-85775-395-X   £19.95

Hope, S.
Hormone replacement therapy: a guide for primary care
Oxford UP 170pp Paperback 1999
0-19-262956-5   £14.99

Jones, R.
General practice: essential facts
Radcliffe Medical 120pp Paperback 1999
1-85775-250-3   £17.95

Kendrick, T.
Prevention of mental illness in primary care
Cambridge UP 414pp Paperback 1996
0-521-57648-2   £35.00

Khot, A.
Practical general practice
Butterworth-Heinemann 256pp 3e. Paperback 1999
0-7506-3462-6 £35.00

Lakhani, M.
Evidence-based audit
Butterworth-Heinemann 160pp Paperback 1998
0-7506-3104-X £16.99

Lawrence, M.
Prevention of cardiovascular disease
Oxford UP 352pp Hardback 1996
0-19-262397-4 £29.95

Lawrence, N.
Handbook of emergencies in general practice
Oxford UP 390pp Paperback 1996
0-19-262545-4 £19.95

Lilley, R.
The PCG team builder
Radcliffe Medical 128pp Paperback 1999
1-85775-308-9 £30.00

Lilley, R.
The PCG toolkit
Radcliffe Medical 160pp 2e. Paperback 1999
1-85775-338-0 £30.00

Loudon, I.
**General practice under the National Health
Service 1948-1997**
Clarendon Press 360pp Hardback 1998
0-19-820675-5 £45.00

Mayon-White, R.
Immunizing children: a practical guide
Radcliffe Medical 104pp Paperback 1998
1-85775-219-8 £14.95

McCormick, A.
Morbidity statistics from general practice
Stationery Office 382pp Paperback 1995
0-11-691610-9 £30.00

McEvoy, P.
Educating the future GP
Radcliffe Medical 328pp 2e. Hardback 1998
1-85775-281-3 £35.00

McPherson, A.
Women's health
Oxford UP 664pp 4e. Paperback 1997
0-19-262750-3 £29.95

McWhinney, I.R.
A textbook of family medicine
Oxford UP Inc 460pp Paperback 1997
0-19-511518-X £29.95

Mead, M.
Tutorials in general practice
Churchill Livingstone 200pp 3e. Paperback 1999
0-443-06197-1 £25.00

Modell, M.
Paediatric problems in general practice
Oxford UP 352pp Paperback 1996
0-19-262512-8 £27.50

Moore, R.
The MRCGP examination book
Royal Col of General 218pp 3e. Paperback 1998
0-85084-241-7 £21.50

Moreton, P.
The very stuff of general practice
Radcliffe Medical 216pp Hardback 1999
1-85775-390-9 £35.00

Moulds, A.
Emergencies in general practice
Petroc Press 256pp 4e. Paperback 1999
1-900603-86-1 £19.95

Neighbour, R.
The inner consultation
Petroc Press 340pp Paperback 1999
1-900603-67-5 £19.95

Neighbour, R.
The inner apprentice
Petroc Press 242pp Paperback 2000
1-900603-04-7 £22.95

O'Dowd, T.
Men's health
Oxford UP 290pp Paperback 1998
0-19-262581-0 £29.50

Palmer, K.T.
Notes for the MRCGP
Blackwell Science USA 336pp 3e. Paperback 1997
0-86542-777-1 £19.95

Pringle, M.
Core values in primary care
BMJ Books 80pp Paperback 1998
0-7279-1268-2 £12.95

Robbins, M.
Medical receptionists and secretaries handbook
Radcliffe Medical 304pp 2e. Paperback 1998
1-85775-249-X £14.99

Rowlands, S.
Managing family planning in general practice
Radcliffe Medical 152pp Paperback 1997
1-85775-205-8 £17.95

Sambandan, S.
Surgery in the surgery
Radcliffe Medical 280pp Paperback 1999
1-85775-284-8 £29.95

Singer, R.
GP commissioning
Radcliffe Medical 176pp Paperback 1997
1-85775-184-1 £19.95

Stacey, E.
Hot topics in general practice
Bios Scientific 416pp 3e.Paperback 2000
1-85996-129-0   £24.95

Stephenson, A.
A textbook of general practice
Arnold 256pp Paperback 1998
0-340-67664-7   £18.99

Van Zwanenberg, T.
Clinical governance and primary care
Radcliffe Medical 200pp Paperback 1999
1-85775-396-8   £21.50

Walshe, K.
Accreditation in primary care
Radcliffe Medical 172pp Paperback 1999
1-85775-322-4   £18.95

Wilkinson, G.
Treating people with anxiety and stress
Radcliffe Medical 264pp Paperback 1999
1-85775-139-6   £19.95

Wilkinson, G.
Treating people with depression
Radcliffe Medical 168pp Paperback 1999
1-85775-391-7   £17.95

GENETICS

Connor, J.M.
Essential medical genetics
Blackwell Science UK 248pp 5e. Paperback 1997
0-86542-666-X   £18.50

Gelehrter, T.D.
The principles of medical genetics
Williams and Wilkins 421pp 2e. Hardback 1998
0-683-03445-6   £19.95

Harper, P.S.
Practical genetic counselling
Butterworth-Heinemann 370pp 5e. Paperback 1998
0-7506-3368-9   £39.50

Jorde, L.B.
Medical genetics
Mosby 352pp 2e. Paperback 1998
0-8151-4608-6   £19.95

King, R.C.
A dictionary of genetics
Oxford UP Inc 448pp 5e. 1997
0-19-509441-7 Hardback   £47.50
0-19-509442-5 Paperback   £23.50

Kingston, H.
ABC of clinical genetics
BMJ Books 84pp 2e. Paperback 1997
0-7279-1101-5   £16.95

McKusick, V.A.
Mendelian inheritance in man
12e. 3 vols Johns Hopkins UP 3792pp
Hardback 1997
0-8018-5742-2   £134.50

Mueller, R.F.
Emery's elements of medical genetics
Churchill Livingstone 376pp 10e. Paperback 1998
0-443-05902-0   £21.95

Rimoin, D.L.
**Emery and Rimoin's principles and practice of
medical genetics**
Churchill Livingstone 2756pp 3e. Hardback 1996
0-443-04851-7   £325.00

Strachan, T.
Human molecular genetics
Bios Scientific 587pp 2e. Paperback 1999
1-85996-202-5   £29.95

GERIATRIC MEDICINE
(See also Community Care)

Allen, S.C.
Medicine in old age
Churchill Livingstone 216pp 4e. Paperback 1998
0-443-05778-8   £15.95

Bennett, G.C.J.
The essentials of health care in old age
Arnold 247pp 2e. Paperback 1995
0-340-61372-6   £14.99

Burns, A.
Assessment scales in old age psychiatry
Martin Dunitz 200pp Paperback 1999
1-85317-562-5   £24.95

Butler, R.
Seminars in old age psychiatry
Gaskell 360pp Paperback 1998
1-901242-21-8   £17.50

Cassel, C.K.
Geriatric medicine
Springer-Verlag NY 960pp 3e. Hardback 1996
0-387-94692-6   £99.00

Coni, N.
Lecture notes on geriatrics
Blackwell Science UK 216pp 5e. Paperback 1997
0-86542-750-X   £14.95

Denham, M.J.
Continuing care for older people
Stanley Thornes 413pp Paperback 1997
0-7487-3182-2   £26.50

Downton, J.H.
Falls in the elderly
Arnold 160pp Paperback 1993
0-340-54848-7   £22.50

Evans, J.G.
Oxford textbook of geriatric medicine
Oxford UP 1008pp 2e. Hardback 2000
0-19-262830-5   £150.00

Gauthier, S.
Clinical diagnosis and management of Alzheimer's disease
Martin Dunitz 400pp 2e. Hardback 1999
1-85317-655-9   £69.95

Iliffe, S.
Health care for older people
BMJ Books 187pp Paperback 1998
0-7279-1192-9   £18.95

Jacoby, R.
Psychiatry in the elderly
Oxford UP 814pp 2e. 1996
0-19-262789-9 Hardback   £99.50
0-19-262788-0 Paperback   £49.50

Mayer, P.P.
Quality care for elderly people
Arnold 312pp Hardback 1997
0-412-61830-3   £55.00

Mulley, G.
Older people at home: practical issues
BMJ Books 147pp Paperback 1998
0-7279-1258-5   £17.95

Pathy, M.S.J.
Principles and practice of geriatric medicine
John Wiley 1688pp 3e. Hardback 1998
0-471-96348-8   £250.00

Philp, I.
Assessing elderly patients
Farrand Press 176pp Paperback 1994
1-85083-034-7   £14.95

Royal Commission on Long Term Care
With respect to old age: long term care - rights and responsibilities (report)
Stationery Office 207pp Paperback 1999
0-10-141922-8   £18.00

Schrier, R.
Geriatric medicine
Blackwell Science USA 969pp 2e. Hardback 1996
0-86542-394-6   £115.00

Shukla, R.B.
Care of the elderly
Stationery Office 145pp 2e. Paperback 1999
0-11-702334-5   £16.95

Sinclair, A.J.
Acute medical illness in old age
Arnold 304pp Hardback 1995
0-412-56920-5   £69.00

Tallis, J.C.
Brocklehurt's textbook of geriatrics and gerontology
Churchill Livingstone 1800pp 5e. Hardback 1998
0-443-05370-7   £155.00

HAEMATOLOGY

Bain, B.J.
Blood cells
Blackwell Science UK 336pp 2e. Paperback 1996
0-632-04155-2   £33.50

Bain, B.J.
Bone marrow pathology
Blackwell Science UK 344pp 2e. Hardback 1996
0-86542-647-3   £79.50

Beutler, E.
William's hematology
McGraw-Hill HPD 1920pp 5e. Hardback 1995
0-07-070386-8   £120.00

Contreras, M.
ABC of transfusion
BMJ Books 91pp 3e. Paperback 1998
0-7279-1209-7   £15.95

Dacie, J.V.
Practical haematology
Churchill Livingstone 608pp 8e. Paperback 1995
0-443-04931-9   £65.00

Daniels, G.
Human blood groups
Blackwell Science USA 768pp Hardback 1995
0-86542-914-6   £89.50

Hoffbrand, A.V.
Essential haematology
Blackwell Science UK 447pp 3e. Paperback 1992
0-632-01954-9   £19.50

Hoffbrand, A.V.
Postgraduate haematology
Butterworth-Heinemann 768pp 4e. Hardback 1997
0-7506-0583-9   £105.00

Hoffbrand, A.V.
Clinical hematology
Mosby 368pp 3e. Hardback 2000
0-7234-3115-9   £129.00

Hoffman, R.
Hematology
Churchill Livingstone 2368pp Hardback 1999
0-443-07954-4   £139.00

Howard, M.R.
Haematology
Churchill Livingstone 120pp Paperback 1997
0-443-05276-X   £17.95

Hughes-Jones, N.C.
Lecture notes on haematology
Blackwell Science UK 283pp 6e. Paperback 1996
0-632-04039-4   £14.95

Lee, G.R.
Wintrobe's clinical hematology
Williams and Wilkins 2680pp 10e. Hardback 1998
0-683-18242-0   £120.00

Mehta, A.B.
Haematology at a glance
Blackwell Science UK 96pp Paperback 2000
0-632-04793-3   £13.95

Mollison, PL.
Blood transfusion in clinical medicine
Blackwell Science UK 784pp 10e. Hardback 1997
0-86542-881-6   £79.50

Nagel, R.L.
Sickle cell anemia
Blackwell Science USA 600pp Hardback 1997
0-86542-060-2   £75.00

Provan, D.
Molecular haematology
Blackwell Science UK 264pp Hardback 1999
0-632-05037-3   £95.00

Provan, D.
Oxford handbook of clinical haematology
Oxford UP 634pp Paperback 1998
0-19-262903-4   £19.95

Provan, D.
Clinical haematology
Butterworth-Heinemann 240pp Paperback 1997
0-7506-2920-7   £27.50

Provan, D.
ABC of clinical haematology
BMJ Books 80pp Paperback 1997
0-7279-1206-2   £16.95

Wood, J.K.
Standard haematology practice 3
Blackwell Science UK 304pp Hardback 1999
0-632-05322-4   £69.50

Wood, K.
Standard haematology practice 2
Blackwell Science UK 304pp Hardback 1994
0-632-03739-3   £49.50

HEALTH ADMINISTRATION
Finance and Health Economics

Department of Health
Public private partnerships in the NHS
Stationery Office Ringbound 153pp 1999
0-11-321865-6   £40.00

Donaldson, C.
Why a national health service?
IPPR Paperback 1998
1-86030-081-2   £4.95

Earl-Slater, A.
Dictionary of health economics
Radcliffe Medical 164pp Paperback 1999
1-85775-337-2   £19.95

Gladstone, D.
How to pay for health care
Institute for the Study of Civil Society 60pp
Paperback 1997
0-255-36397-4   £6.00

Le Grand, J.
Learning the NHS internal markets
King's Fund 207pp Paperback 1998
1-85717-215-9   £15.99

McCrone, P.
Understanding health economics
Open UP 160pp Paperback 1998
0-335-20592-5   £16.99

Prowle, M.
Health Service finance: an introduction
Certified Accountant 4e.Paperback 1997
1-85908-121-5   £19.50

Smith, C.
Making sense of the private finance initiative
Radcliffe Medical 232pp Paperback 1999
1-85775-381-X   £27.50

Smith, P.C.
Reforming markets in health care
Open UP 308pp Paperback 2000
0-335-20461-9   £19.99

HEALTH ADMINISTRATION
General Texts

Baggott, R.
Health and health care in Britain
Macmillan Press 384pp 2e. Paperback 1998
0-333-69476-7   £16.99

Baker, M.
Making sense of the NHS White Papers
Radcliffe Medical 264pp 2e. Paperback 1999
1-85775-460-3   £18.95

Brooks, B.
Managing change in the NHS
Open UP 144pp Paperback 1999
0-335-20593-3   £18.99

Busfield, J.
Health and health care in modern Britain
Oxford UP 180pp Paperback 2000
0-19-878123-7   £12.99

Department of Health
The new NHS: modern and dependable
Stationery Office 86pp Paperback 1997
0-10-138072-0   £12.50

Directory of Hospitals and Trusts
Informa Healthcare 1142pp Paperback 2000
1-85978-569-7   £99.00

Ham, C.
The politics of NHS reform 1988-97
King's Fund 78pp Paperback 2000
1-85717-417-8   £14.99

Ham, C.
Health policy in Britain
Macmillan Press 256pp Paperback 1999
0-333-76407-2   £14.99

Harrison, A.
Health care UK 2000 - spring
(three issues per year) King's Fund 264pp
Paperback 2000
1-85717-413-5   £9.99

Harrison, A.
The NHS: facing the future
King's Fund 354pp Paperback 2000
1-85717-219-1   £17.99

Hutton, W.
New life for health
Vintage Paperback 142pp Paperback 2000
0-09-928575-4   £4.99

Jones, T.
Structure of the National Health Service
Pub Initiatives 2e. Paperback 1998
1-873839-17-0   £14.95

Leathard, A.
Healthcare provision: past, present and future
Stanley Thornes 240pp Paperback 2000
0-7487-3354-X   £22.50

Levitt, R.
The re-organised National Health Service
Stanley Thornes 278pp 6e. Paperback 1999
0-7487-3894-0   £22.50

Ling, T.
Reforming healthcare by consent
Radcliffe Medical 248pp Paperback 1998
1-85775-321-6   £22.50

Macpherson, G.
Our NHS: a celebration of 50 years
BMJ Books 242pp Hardback 1998
0-7279-1279-8   £25.00

Marinker, M.
Clinical futures
BMJ Books 230pp Paperback 1998
0-7279-1231-3   £19.95

Morgan, O.
Who cares? The great British health debate
Radcliffe Medical 240pp Paperback 1998
1-85775-243-0   £18.95

Paton, C.
Competition and planning in the National Health Service
Stanley Thornes 192pp 2e. Paperback 1998
0-7487-3307-8   £18.50

Pollard, S.
A question of choice
Social Market Fdn Paperback 1999
1-874097-59-3   £10.00

Ranade, W.
A future for the NHS?
Longman Higher Ed 246pp 2e. Paperback 1997
0-582-28993-9   £17.99

Salter, B.
The politics of change in the health service
Palgrave 272pp Paperback 1998
0-333-65641-5   £16.99

Spurgeon, P.
The new face of the NHS
Royal Soc Medicine 306pp 2e. Paperback 1998
0-443-05969-1   £17.99

Timmins, N.
The five giants of the NHS
Fontana 600pp Paperback 1996
0-00-686318-3   £10.99

Wellard's NHS handbook 2000/2001
JMH Publishing 300pp Paperback 2000
0-953368-43-2   £45.00

HEALTH ADMINISTRATION
Management

Austin, N.
The clinical directorate
Radcliffe Medical 174pp Paperback 1997
1-85775-037-3   £19.95

Cropper, S.
Enhancing Health Services management
Open UP 256pp Paperback 1997
0-335-19634-9 £22.50

Debell, B.
Conciliation and mediation in the NHS
Radcliffe Medical 104pp Paperback 1997
1-85775-231-7 £17.95

Dopson, S.
Managing ambiguity and change
Macmillan Press 184pp Paperback 1997
0-333-66906-1 £20.00

Ham, C.
Management and competition in the NHS
Radcliffe Medical 96pp 2e. Paperback 1997
1-85775-104-3 £17.95

Holdaway, K.
The healthcare management handbook
Kogan Page 406pp 2e. Paperback 1997
0-7494-2155-X £20.00

Iles, V.
Really managing health care
Open UP 208pp Paperback 1997
0-335-19414-1 £18.99

Meads, G.
Relationships in today's NHS
Royal Soc Medicine Paperback 1999
1-85315-438-5 £17.50

Riley, J.
Helping doctors who manage
King's Fund 168pp Paperback 1998
1-85717-147-0 £14.99

Roberts, K.
Project management for health care professionals
Butterworth-Heinemann 224pp Paperback 1998
0-7506-3405-7 £16.99

Smith, J.
Health management information systems
Open UP 356pp Paperback 1999
0-335-20565-8 £22.50

Soothill, K.
Interprofessional relations in health care
Arnold 376pp Paperback 1994
0-340-59806-9 £16.99

Young, A.E.
The medical manager
BMJ Books 304pp Paperback 1999
0-7279-1376-X £25.00

HEALTH ADMINISTRATION
Quality, Audit and Clinical Governance

Baker, R.
Implementing change in clinical audit
John Wiley 200pp Paperback 1999
0-471-98257-1 £19.99

Bullivant, J.
Benchmarking for best value in the NHS
FT Pharmaceuticals 152pp 1998
1-86067-353-8 £95.00

Davies, H.T.O.
Managing quality: strategic issues in health care management
Ashgate 256pp Hardback 1999
0-7546-1004-7 £39.95

Department of Health
A first class service: quality in the new NHS
Department of Health 86pp Paperback 1998
No ISBN gratis

Enthoven, A.C.
In pursuit of an improving NHS
Nuffield Trust 126pp Hardback 1999
1-902089-37-5 £15.00

Gillies, A.
Improving the quality of patient care
John Wiley 230pp Paperback 1997
0-471-96647-9 £19.99

Heard , S.
Clinical governance
Arnold 192pp Paperback 2000
0-340-76013-3 £17.99

Institute of Health Services Management:
Clinical governance: a toolkit for managers
Ashgate 112pp 1999
0-7546-1004-7 £39.95

Jenkinson, C.
Assessment and evaluation of health and medical care
Open UP 176pp Paperback 1997
0-335-19705-1 £16.99

Lilley, R.
Making sense of clinical governance
Radcliffe Medical 166pp Paperback 1999
1-85775-425-5 £30.00

Lugon, M.
Clinical governance: making it happen
Royal Soc Med 232pp Paperback 1999
1-85315-383-4 £17.50

Miles, A.
NICE, CHI and the NHS reform
Aesculapius Med Press Paperback 2000
1-903044-06-5   £19.99

Morton-Cooper, A.
Excellence in health care management
Blackwell Science UK 264pp Paperback 1997
0-632-04032-7   £16.99

Ovretveit, J.
Evaluating health interventions
Open UP 335pp Paperback 1998
0-335-19964-X   £19.99

Parsley, K.
Quality improvement in nursing and healthcare
Stanley Thornes 299pp 2e. Paperback 1998
0-7487-3355-8   £23.50

Powell, M.A.
Evaluating the National Health Service
Open UP 224pp Paperback 1997
0-335-19530-X   £15.99

Scotland, A.
Clinical governance: one year on
Quay Books 200pp Paperback 2000
1-85642-185-6   £12.99

Swage, T.
Clinical governance in healthcare practice
Butterworth-Heinemann 256pp Paperback 2000
0-7506-4453-2   £17.99

HEALTH PROMOTION

Bright, J.S.
Health promotion in clinical practice
Bailliere Tindall 256pp Paperback 1996
1-873853-41-6   £14.95

Davies, J.K.
Quality, evidence and effectiveness in health promotion
Routledge 240pp 1998
0-415-17966-1 Hardback   £55.00
0-415-17967-X Paperback   £15.99

Downie, R.S.
Health promotion
Oxford UP 232pp Paperback 1996
0-19-262591-8   £14.95

Evans, D.
Assuring quality in health promotion (computer disc version)
Health Education Mixed-media pack 1994
0-7521-0245-1   £18.00

Ewles, L.
Promoting health
Bailliere Tindall 352pp 4e. Paperback 1998
0-7020-2308-6   £16.95

Jones, L.
The challenge of promoting health
Macmillan Press 320pp 1997
0-333-68173-8 Hardback   £45.00
0-333-68174-6 Paperback   £14.99

Kemm, J.
Health promotion: theory and practice
Macmillan Press 383pp Paperback 1995
0-333-57769-8   £15.50

Lask, S.
Promoting the health of the nation
Churchill Livingstone 264pp Paperback 1997
0-443-05225-5   £31.95

Naidoo, J.
Health promotion
Bailliere Tindall 412pp 2e. Paperback 2000
0-7020-2448-1   £17.95

Pike, S.
Health promotion for all
Churchill Livingstone 220pp Paperback 1995
0-443-05089-9   £18.95

Scott, D.
Evaluating health promotion
Stanley Thornes 182pp Paperback 1998
0-7487-3313-2   £19.50

Scriven, A.
Health promotion
Macmillan Press 264pp Paperback 1996
0-333-64497-2   £15.50

Seedhouse, D.
Health promotion
John Wiley Litd 212pp Paperback 1996
0-471-93910-2   £19.99

Sidell, M.
Debates and dilemmas in promoting health
Macmillan Press 400pp 1997
0-333-69416-3 Hardback   £47.50
0-333-69417-1 Paperback   £15.99

Simnett, I.
Evidence-based health promotion
John Wiley 448pp Paperback 1999
0-471-97851-5   £29.95

Simnett, K.I.
Managing health promotion
John Wiley 248pp 1995
0-471-95814-X Hardback   £24.95
0-19-263169-1 Paperback   £17.95

Webb, P.
Health promotion and patient education
Stanley Thornes 330pp Paperback 1997
0-7487-3564-X   £21.00

IMMUNOLOGY & ALLERGY

Chapel, H.
Essentials of clinical immunology
Blackwell Science UK 400pp 4e. Paperback 1999
0-632-04972-3   £24.95

Department of Health
Immunisation against infectious diseases
Stationery Office 230pp Paperback 1995
0-11-321815-X   £6.95

Durham, S.
ABC of allergies
BMJ Books 72pp Paperback 1998
0-7279-1236-4   £14.95

Holgate, S.T.
Allergy
Mosby 352pp 2e. Paperback 2000
0-7234-3066-7   £59.95

Janeway, C.A.
Immunobiology
Churchill Livingstone 600pp 4e. 1999
0-443-06275-7 Paperback   £29.95
0-443-06421-0 CD-ROM   £76.38

Mackett, M.
Human vaccines and vaccination
Bios Scientific 232pp Paperback 1995
1-872748-77-5   £19.95

Male, D.K.
Advanced immunology
Mosby 273pp 3e. Hardback 1996
0-7234-2059-9   £35.95

Mayon-White, R.
Immunizing children: a practical guide
Radcliffe Medical 104pp 2e. Paperback 1998
1-85775-219-8   £14.95

Mygind, N.
Essential allergy
Blackwell Science UK 448pp 2e. Hardback 1995
0-632-03645-1   £29.50

Peakman, M.
Basic and clinical immunology
Churchill Livingstone 320pp Paperback 1997
0-443-04672-7   £21.95

Playfair, J.H.L.
Infection and immunity
Oxford UP 160pp Paperback 1995
0-19-854925-3   £14.95

Reeves, G.
Lecture notes on immunology .
Blackwell Science UK 280pp 4e. Paperback 2000
0-632-05636-3   £14.95

Roitt, I.M.
Roitt's essential immunology
Blackwell Science UK 496pp 9e. Paperback 1997
0-86542-729-1   £19.95

Roitt, I.
Immunology
Mosby 416pp 5e. Paperback 1997
0-7234-2918-9   £26.95

Spickett, G.
Oxford handbook of clinical immunology
Oxford UP 732pp Paperback 1999
0-19-262721-X   £19.95

Stites, D.P.
Medical immunology
Appleton and Lange 890pp 9e. Paperback 1997
0-8385-6278-7   £31.00

Weir, D.M.
Handbook of experimental immunology
4 vols Blackwell Science USA 2426pp 5e.
Hardback 1997
0-86542-421-7   £450.00

Weir, D.M.
Immunology
Churchill Liv 368pp 8e. Paperback 1997
0-443-05452-5   £19.95

INFECTIOUS DISEASES
(See also Immunology & Allergy, Microbiology, Sexually Transmitted Diseases)

Armstrong, D.
Infectious diseases
2 vols Mosby 2040pp Hardback 1999
0-7234-2328-8   £250.00

Ayliffe, G.A.J.
Control of hospital infection
Arnold 416pp 4e. Hardback 2000
0-340-75911-9   £45.00

Ayliffe, G.A.J.
Hospital acquired infection
Butterworth-Heinemann 208pp 3e. Paperback 1999
0-7506-2105-2   £18.99

Ball, A.P.
Infectious diseases
Churchill Liv 132pp 2e. Paperback 2000
0-443-05883-0   £9.50

Bannister, B.
Infectious diseases
Blackwell Science UK 448pp 2e. Paperback 2000
0-632-05319-4 £29.50

Collins, C.H.
Laboratory-acquired infections
Butterworth-Heinemann 288pp 4e. Hardback 1998
0-7506-4023-5 £45.00

Conlon, C.
Color atlas and text of infectious diseases
Mosby 320pp Paperback 2000
0-7234-2434-9 £28.95

Damani, N.N.
Manual of infection control procedures
Greenwich Medical 234pp Paperback 1997
1-900151-28-6 £22.50

Emond, R.T.D.
Colour atlas of infectious diseases
Mosby 436pp 3e. Paperback 1994
0-7234-2127-7 £21.95

Mandal, B.K.
Lecture notes on infectious diseases
Blackwell Science UK 368pp 5e. Paperback 1995
0-632-03351-7 £16.95

Mandell, G.L.
Principles and practice of infectious diseases
Churchill Livingstone 3536pp 5e. Hardback 1999
0-443-07593-X £199.00

Mercier, C.
Infection control: hospital and community
Stanley Thornes 235pp Paperback 1997
0-7487-3319-1 £18.00

Mims, C.
The pathogenesis of infectious disease
Academic Press 416pp 5e. Paperback 2000
0-12-498265-4 £29.95

Russell, A.D.
Principles and practice of disinfection, preservation and sterilisation
Blackwell Science UK 780pp 3e. Hardback 1998
0-632-04194-3 £85.00

Shulman, S.T.
The biologic and clinical basis of infectious diseases
W B Saunders 659pp 5e. Paperback 1996
0-7216-5948-9 £44.95

Southgate, L.
Infection
Oxford UP 476pp Paperback 1997
0-19-262092-4 £29.95

Wilks, D.
The infectious disease manual
Blackwell Science USA 384pp Paperback 1995
0-86542-844-1 £19.95

INFERTILITY

Balen, A.
Infertility in practice
Churchill Livingstone 400pp Paperback 1997
0-443-05356-1 £43.95

Barratt, C.L.R.
Male fertility and infertility
Cambridge UP 286pp Hardback 1999
0-521-62375-8 £45.00

Burns, L.H.
Infertility counselling
Parthenon 408pp Hardback 1998
1-85070-924-6 £38.00

Chambers, R.
Fertility problems
Radcliffe Medical 112pp Paperback 1999
1-85775-302-X £17.95

Elder, K.
In vitro fertilization
Cambridge UP 322pp 2e. Paperback 2000
0-521-77863-8 £34.95

Jansen, R.
Overcoming infertility
W H Freeman 474pp Paperback 1998
0-7167-3302-1 £12.95

Rainsbury, P.A.
Practical guide to reproductive medicine
Parthenon 250pp Hardback 1997
1-85070-727-8 £48.00

Royal College of Obstetricians and Gynaecologists
The management of infertility in secondary care
Royal College of Obs 148pp Paperback 1998
1-900364-16-6 £17.00

Seibel, M.
Infertility: a comprehensive text
Appleton and Lange 670pp Hardback 1997
0-8385-4258-1 £85.00

Templeton, A.
Evidence-based fertility treatment
Royal College of Obstetricians and Gynaecologists
Hardback 1998
1-900364-10-7 £65.00

LEGISLATION
(See also Forensic Medicine & Medical Law)
Commentaries

Department of Health
Mental Health Act 1983: code of practice
Stationery Office 176pp 3e. Paperback 1999
0-11-322111-8 £7.50

Allen, N.
Making sense of the Children Act
John Wiley 298pp 3e. Paperback 1998
0-471-97831-0 £16.99

Cornish, G.P.
Copyright: interpreting the law for libraries, archives and information services
Library Assoc Publ 193pp 3e. Paperback 1999
1-85604-344-4 £19.95

Dimond, B.
Mental Health (patients in the community) Act 1995: introductory guide
Quay Books 100pp Paperback 1997
1-85642-012-4 £10.99

Dolan, B.
The Mental Health Act, explained
Stationery Office 250pp Paperback 1999
0-11-702345-0 £25.00

Doyle, B.
Disability discrimination: law and practice
Family Law 3e. Paperback 2000
0-85308-568-4 £39.00

Gooding, C.
Blackstone's guide to the Disability Discrimination Act 1995
Blackstone Press 138pp Paperback1996
1-85431-499-8 £14.95

Jones, R.
Mental Health Act manual
Sweet & Maxwell 717pp 6e. Paperback 1999
0-421-67480-6 £46.00

Lee, R.G.
Human fertilisation and embryology
Blackstone Press Paperback 2000
1-84174-119-1 £25.00

Mitchels, B.
Child care and protection law and practice
Cavendish Publishing 152pp 2e. Paperback 1996
1-85941-292-0 £15.95

Norman, S.
Copyright in health libraries
Library Assoc Publ 104pp 3e. Paperback 1999
1-85604-323-1 £9.95

Ryan, M.
The Children Act 1989: putting it into practice
Arena 272pp 2e. Paperback 1999
1-85742-433-6 £16.95

Acts of Parliament 1997-1999 (for older Acts see the 3rd edition of the Core Collection 1997)

Community Care (Residential Accommodation) Act 1998
Stationery Office Paperback 1998
0-10-541998-2 £1.10

Data Protection Act 1998
Stationery Office 86pp Paperback 1998
0-10-542998-8 £10.30

Disability Rights Commission Act 1999
Stationery Office Paperback 1999
0-10-541799-8 £5.00

The Health Act 1999
Stationery Office 114pp Paperback 1999
0-10-540899-9 £12.35

National Health Service (Primary Care) Act 1997
Stationery Office 66pp Paperback 1997
0-10-544697-1 £8.40

National Health Service (Private Finance) Act 1997
Stationery Office Paperback 1997
0-10-545697-7 £0.65

Nurses, Midwives and Health Visitors Act 1997
Stationery Office Paperback 1997
0-10-542497-8 £4.85

MEDICAL ETHICS

Bloch, S.
Psychiatric ethics
Oxford UP 562pp Paperback 1999
0-19-262899-2 £34.50

Boyd, K.M.
New dictionary of medical ethics
BMJ Books 304pp Paperback 1997
0-7279-1001-9 £22.00

British Medical Association
Withholding and withdrawing life-prolonging medical treatment
BMJ Books 95pp Paperback 1999
0-7279-1456-1 £9.95

The first UK National Paediatric Formulary

Medicines for Children

The essential reference tool for health libraries and information units.

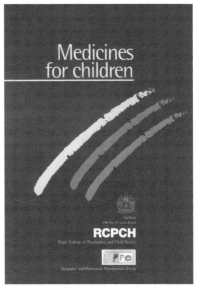

- Aims to represent current best practice, based on the authority of experts.
- Overseen by a formulary advisory group consisting of members of the RCPCH and NPPG and was funded by the Nuffield Foundation.
- Extensively peer reviewed.

Has three main parts:

- Therapeutic guidelines providing information on which medicines to prescribe by clinical need.
- Drug monographs containing information on drugs given to children, both licenced and unlicenced.
- Dietary section of ACBS products presented in tabular form.

Aimed at

- ✔ **Clinicians** who prescribe drugs for children;
- ✔ **Pharmacists** who dispense or advise about drugs for children;
- ✔ **Dietitians** who recommend special feeds in children;
- ✔ **General Practitioners** and **carers** who administer drugs to children.

Published by the Royal College of Paediatrics and Child Health (RCPCH)

"...provides prescribing advice for more than 300 medicines used in children, whether or not they hold a licence for paediatric use"
Hospital Doctor

"...the first comprehensive study on drugs used to treat babies and children"
Daily Mail

"...a guide that seeks to give authoritative backing for the use of drugs not licensed for use on children so that all doctors will prescribe them if necessary."
Times

Medicines for Children – 1999 Edition
ISBN 1900954389   £48.95

International Booksellers

BMBC Ltd. Headlands Business Park Ringwood, Hampshire, BH24 3PB Tel: 01425 471160 Fax: 01425 471525

e-mail: directbooks@bmbc.com   www.bmbc.com

British Medical Association
Medical ethics today
BMA Professional 385pp Paperback 1993
0-7279-0817-0   £12.95

Campbell, A.
Medical ethics
Oxford UP Aus & NZ 238pp Paperback 1997
0-19-558350-7   £19.95

Downie, R.S.
Healthy respect: ethics in health care
Oxford UP 310pp 2e. Paperback 1994
0-19-262408-3   £16.50

Goodman, K.
Ethics, computing and medicine
Cambridge UP 192pp Paperback 1998
0-521-46905-8   £17.95

Marteau, T.
The troubled helix
Cambridge UP 380pp Paperback 1999
0-521-58612-7   £19.95

Mason, J.K.
Law and medical ethics
5e. Butterworths Law 628pp Paperback 1999
0-406-89636-4   £19.95

McCullough, L.B.
Surgical ethics
Oxford UP 416pp Hardback 1998
0-19-510347-5   £37.50

New, B.
Rationing: talk and action in health care
BMJ Books 280pp Paperback 1997
0-7279-1180-5   £25.00

Palmer, M.
Moral problems in medicine
Lutterworth Press 190pp Paperback 1999
0-7188-2978-6   £14.50

Seedhouse, D.
Ethics: the heart of health care
John Wiley Ltd 250pp 2e. Hardback 1998
0-471-97592-3   £16.99

Singleton, J.
Ethical foundations of health care
Mosby 224pp Paperback 1995
0-7234-1873-X   £11.00

Smith, T.
Ethics in medical research: a handbook of good practice
Cambridge UP 422pp Paperback 1999
0-521-62619-6   £29.95

Warnock, M.
An intelligent person's guide to ethics
Duckworth 128pp Paperback 1998
0-7156-2841-0   £12.95

MEDICAL WRITING & RESEARCH

Albert, T.
A-Z of medical writing
BMJ Books 150pp Paperback 2000
0-7279-1487-1   £15.00

Albert, T.
Winning the publications game
Radcliffe Medical 120pp Paperback 2000
1-85775-471-9   £18.95

Baker, M.
Research and development for the NHS
Radcliffe Medical 184pp 2e. Paperback 1998
1-85775-213-9   £19.95

Bowling, A.
Research methods in health
Open UP 442pp Paperback 1997
0-335-19885-6   £18.99

Briscoe, M.H.
Preparing scientific illustrations
Springer-Verlag NY 215pp 2e. Paperback 1996
0-387-94581-4   £17.00

Crombie, I.K.
Research into health care
John Wiley Ltd 302pp Paperback 1996
0-471-96259-7   £27.50

Day, R.A.
How to write and publish a scientific paper
Cambridge UP 275pp 5e. Paperback 1998
0-521-65879-9   £12.95

Department of Health
Supporting research and development in the NHS
Stationery Office 90pp Paperback 1994
0-11-321831-1   £5.95

Fraser, J.
How to publish in biomedicine
Radcliffe Medical 232pp Paperback 1997
1-85775-193-0   £17.95

Goodman, N.W.
Medical writing
Cambridge UP 239pp 2e. Paperback 1997
0-521-49876-7   £19.95

Hadfield-Law, L.
Effective presentations for healthcare professionals
Butterworth-Heinemann 224pp Paperback 1999
0-7506-3843-5   £14.99

Hall, G.M.
How to write a paper
BMJ Books 157pp 2e. Paperback 1998
0-7279-1234-8   £13.95

Huth, E.
Scientific style and format
Cambridge UP 841pp 6e. Hardback 1995
0-521-47154-0   £24.95

Iverson, C.
American Medical Association manual of style
Williams and Wilkins 660pp 9e. Hardback 1998
0-683-40206-4   £25.00

Matthews, J.R.
Successful scientific writing
Cambridge UP 292pp 2e. Paperback 2000
0-521-78962-1   £15.95

Murrell, G.
Research in medicine
Cambridge UP 136pp 2e. Paperback 1999
0-521-62670-6   £12.95

Pope, C.
Qualitative research in health care
BMJ Books 144pp 2e. Hardback 1999
0-7279-1396-4   £14.95

Whimster, W.F.
Biomedical research: how to plan, publish and present it
Springer-Verlag Berl 456pp 2e. Paperback 1997
3-540-19876-8   £12.95

MEDICINE (GENERAL)
(See also Diagnosis & Clinical Methods)

Andreoli, T.E.
Cecil: Essentials of medicine
W B Saunders 1024pp 4e. Paperback 1997
0-7216-6697-3   £34.95

Axford, J.S.
Medicine
Blackwell Science UK 1280pp Paperback 1996
0-632-02707-X   £25.95

Burton, J.L.
Aids to postgraduate medicine
Churchill Liv 259pp 6e. Paperback 1994
0-443-04913-0   £18.95

Burton, J.L.
Aids to undergraduate medicine
Churchill Liv 160pp 6e. Paperback 1997
0-443-05692-7   £13.95

Collier, J.
Oxford handbook of clinical specialties
Oxford UP 864pp 5e. Plastic-reinforced paper 1999
0-19-262943-3   £15.95

Davies, I.J.T.
Postgraduate medicine
Arnold 640pp 6e. Paperback 2000
0-340-76128-8   £29.99

Donald, A.K.
The hands-on guide for house officers
Blackwell Science USA 256pp Paperback 1996
0-86542-921-9   £12.95

Fauci, A.
Harrison's principles of internal medicine
McGraw-Hill HPD 2688pp 14e. Hardback 1997
0-07-020291-5 (In 1 vol)   £81.99
0-07-912013-X (In 2 vols)   £97.99
0-07-135029-2 CD-ROM   £149.21

Forbes, C.D.
Colour atlas and text of clinical medicine
Mosby 576pp 2e. Paperback 1997
0-7234-2198-6   £31.95
0-7234-2795-X CD-ROM   £62.22

Goldman, L.
Cecil Textbook of medicine
W B Saunders 2400pp 21e. Hardback 2000
0-7216-7996-X   £75.00

Haslett, C.
Davidson's principles and practice of medicine
Churchill Liv 1188pp 18e. Paperback 1999
0-443-05944-6   £29.95

Hope, R.A.
Oxford handbook of clinical medicine
Oxford UP 850pp 4e. Plastic-reinforced paper 1998
0-19-262783-X   £14.95

Jones, J.V.
Essential medicine
Churchill Liv 560pp 2e. Paperback 1998
0-443-05811-3   £16.95

Kumar, P.
Clinical medicine
W B Saunders 1352pp 4e. Paperback 1998
0-7020-2019-2   £32.95

Kumar, P.
Acute general medicine: the essentials
Reed Business Information 500pp Paperback 2000
1-873207-02-6   £35.00

Ledingham, J.
Concise Oxford textbook of medicine
Oxford UP 2000pp Hardback 2000
0-19-262870-4   £49.50

McHardy, K.C.
Illustrated signs in clinical medicine
Churchill Liv 168pp Paperback 1997
0-443-05545-9   £16.95

Mitchell, I.
The practical house officer
Blackwell Science UK 352pp 2e. Paperback 1997
0-86542-769-0   £14.95

O'Neill, P.A.
Medicine
Churchill Liv 399pp Paperback 1997
0-443-05078-3   £16.95

Rubenstein, D.
Lecture notes on clinical medicine
Blackwell Science UK 512pp 5e. Paperback 1997
0-86542-925-1   £14.95

Souhami, R.L.
Textbook of medicine
Churchill Liv 1232pp 3e. Paperback 1997
0-443-05592-0   £38.95

Stein, J.H.
Internal medicine
Mosby 2515pp 5e. Hardback 1998
0-8151-8698-3   £69.00
0-323-00372-9 CD-ROM   £123.38

Weatherall, D.J.
Oxford textbook of medicine
3 vols Oxford UP 5024pp 3e. Hardback 1995
0-19-262140-8   £195.00
0-19-268429-9 CD-ROM   £217.38

Zatouroff, M.
Color atlas of physical signs in general medicine
Mosby 448pp 1996
0-7234-2326-1 Hardback   £46.95
0-7234-2587-6 Paperback   £21.95

MICROBIOLOGY
(See also Infectious Diseases, Pharmacology & Toxicology)

Boyd, R.F.
Basic medical microbiology
Williams and Wilkins 768pp 5e. Hardback 1995
0-316-10445-0   £32.00

Brooks, G.F.
Jawetz, Melnick and Adelberg's medical microbiology
Appleton and Lange 752pp 21e. Paperback 1998
0-8385-6316-3   £29.99

Collee, J.G.
Practical medical microbiology
Churchill Liv 978pp 14e. Hardback 1996
0-443-04721-9   £110.00

Collier, L.
Human virology
Oxford UP 224pp 2e. Paperback 2000
0-19-262820-8   £24.95

Collier, L.H.
Topley and Wilson's microbiology and microbial infections
6 vols Arnold 5624pp 9e. 1997
0-340-61470-6 Hardback   £995.00
0-340-70015-7 (Hardback and CD-ROM)   £1,169.13

Collins, C.H.
Collins and Lyne's microbiological methods
Butterworth-Heinemann 440pp 7e. Paperback 1995
0-7506-0653-3   £42.50

Elliott, T.S.J.
Lecture notes on medical microbiology
Blackwell Science UK 352pp 3e. Paperback 1997
0-632-02446-1   £14.95

Emmerson, M.
Principles and practice of clinical bacteriology
John Wiley Ltd 818pp Hardback 1997
0-471-93617-0   £135.00

Forbes, B.A.
Bailey & Scott's diagnostic microbiology
Mosby 960pp 10e. Hardback 1998
0-8151-2535-6   £44.95

Gillespie, S.
Medical microbiology illustrated
Butterworth-Heinemann 304pp Paperback 1998
0-7506-4415-X   £15.99

Greenwood, D.
Medical microbiology
Churchill Liv 690pp 15e. Paperback 1997
0-443-05454-1   £31.95

Hart, C.T.
Medical microbiology
Mosby 320pp Paperback 1996
0-7234-2322-9   £21.95

Inglis, T.J.J.
Microbiology and infection
Churchill Liv 256pp Paperback 1996
0-443-05034-1   £16.95

Mims, C.
Medical microbiology
Mosby 2e. Paperback 1998
0-7234-2781-X   £31.95

Murray, P.R.
Manual of clinical microbiology
Blackwell Science UK 1800pp 7e. 1999
1-55581-126-4 Hardback   £98.00
0-8151-9035-2 Paperback   £25.95

Richardson, M.
Fungal infection: diagnosis and management
Blackwell Science UK 272pp 2e. Paperback 1997
0-86542-724-0 £22.50

Shanson, D.C.
Microbiology in clinical practice
Butterworth-Heinemann 560pp 3e. Paperback 1998
0-7506-3110-4 £29.99

Sleigh, J.D.
Notes on medical bacteriology
Churchill Liv 488pp 5e. Paperback 1998
0-443-05847-4 £17.95

Timbury, M.C.
Notes on medical virology
Churchill Liv 208pp 11e. Paperback 1997
0-443-05845-8 £12.95

Zuckerman, A.J.
Principles and practice of clinical virology
John Wiley Ltd 800pp 4e. Hardback 1999
0-471-97340-8 £165.00

NEUROLOGY & NEUROSURGERY

Adams, R.D.
Principles of neurology
McGraw-Hill USA 1440pp 6e. 1997
0-07-067439-6 Hardback £67.99
0-07-864230-2 CD-ROM £113.99

Bigner, D.D.
Russell and Rubinstein's pathology of tumors of the nervous system
Arnold 1424pp 6e. Hardback 1998
0-340-58113-1 £265.00

Birch, R.
Surgical disorders of the peripheral nerves
Churchill Liv 560pp Hardback 1998
0-443-04443-0 £100.00

Bradley, W.G.
Neurology in clinical practice
Butterworth-Heinemann 326pp 3e. Hardback 1999
0-7506-9973-6 £295.00

Compston, D.A.S.
McAlpine's multiple sclerosis
Churchill Liv 700pp 3e. Hardback 1998
0-443-05008-2 £105.00

Crockard, A.
Neurosurgery
Blackwell Science UK 1440pp 3e. Hardback 1999
0-632-04838-7 £285.00

Donaghy, M.
Neurology
Oxford UP 228pp Paperback 1997
0-19-262795-3 £16.95

Ebrahim, S.
Stroke
Oxford UP 356pp 2e. Paperback 1999
0-19-263075-X £29.50

Ellis, S.
Essentials of clinical neurology
Butterworth-Heinemann 256pp 2e. Paperback 1997
0-7506-3343-3 £17.50

Fuller, G.
Neurological examination made easy
Churchill Liv 232pp 2e. Paperback 1998
0-443-06166-1 £13.50

Fuller, G.
Neurology
Churchill Liv 136pp Paperback 1999
0-443-05374-X £18.95

Gazzaniga, M.S.
The new cognitive neurosciences
The MIT Press 1434pp 2e. Hardback 2000
0-262-07195-9 £80.95

Gilroy, J.
Basic neurology
McGraw-Hill HPD 368pp 3e. Paperback 1999
0-07-105467-7 £30.99

Ginsberg, L.
Lecture notes on neurology
Blackwell Science UK 192pp 7e. Paperback 1999
0-632-04827-1 £14.95

Graham, D.I.
Greenfield's neuropathology
Arnold 2288pp 6e. Hardback 1997
0-340-59809-3 £375.00

Grundy, D.
ABC of spinal cord injury
BMJ Books 80pp Paperback 1996
0-7279-1049-3 £13.95

Harrison, M.J.G.
Clinical skills in neurology
Butterworth-Heinemann 176pp Paperback 1996
0-7506-2520-1 £16.99

Hopkins, A.
Epilepsy
Arnold 696pp 2e. Hardback 1995
0-412-54330-3 £125.00

Hopkins, A.
Epilepsy: the facts
Oxford Paperbacks 168pp 3e. Paperback 1996
0-19-262548-9 £9.99

Hughes, R.A.C.
Neurological emergencies
BMJ Books 250pp 3e. Paperback 2000
0-7279-1405-7 £25.00

Hughes, R.A.C.
Neurological investigations
BMJ Books 250pp Hardback 1997
0-7279-1080-9 £50.00

Kandel, E.J.
Principles of neural science
Appleton and Lange 1568pp 4e. Hardback 1999
0-8385-7701-6 £55.99

Kaye, A.H.
Essential neurosurgery
Churchill Liv 448pp 2e. Paperback 1996
0-443-05347-2 £29.95

Kaye, A.H.
Operative neurosurgery
2 vols Churchill Liv 2496pp Hardback 1999
0-443-05827-X £300.00

Lance, J.W.
Mechanism and management of headache
Butterworth-Heinemann 6e. Hardback 2000
0-7506-4935-6 £25.00

Lindsay, K.W.
Neurology and neurosurgery illustrated
Churchill Liv 576pp 3e. Paperback 1997
0-443-05061-9 £32.95

Marsden, C.D.
Clinical neurology
Arnold 464pp 2e. Paperback 1998
0-340-64611-X £35.00

Park, G.
The management of acute pain
Oxford UP 208pp Paperback 2000
0-19-262467-9 £21.95

Patten, J.P.
Neurological differential diagnosis
Springer-Verlag Berl 465pp 2e. Hardback 1995
3-540-19937-3 £39.50

Perkin, G.D.
Mosby's colour atlas and text of neurology
Mosby 320pp Paperback 1997
0-7234-2497-7 £26.95

Rosenberg, R.N.
Atlas of clinical neurology
Butterworth-Heinemann 400pp Hardback 1998
0-7506-9922-1 £100.00

Rowland, L.P.
Merritt's textbook of neurology
Williams and Wilkins 1000pp Hardback 1995
0-683-07400-8 £75.00

Wall, P.D.
Textbook of pain.
Churchill Liv 1600pp 4e. Hardback 1999
0-443-06252-8 £175.00

Warlow, C.P.
Stroke
Blackwell Science UK 672pp Paperback 1997
0-632-05005-5 £59.50

Wilkinson, I.M.S.
Essential neurology.
Blackwell Science UK 272pp 3e. Paperback 1999
0-86542-854-9 £19.95

NUTRITION & DIETETICS

Abraham, S.
Eating disorders
Oxford UP 254pp Paperback 1996
0-19-262759-7 £8.99

Barker, H.M.
Nutrition and dietetics for health care
Churchill Liv 308pp 9e.Paperback 1996
0-443-05252-2 £21.00

Basu, T.K.
Vitamins in human health and disease
CAB International 368pp Paperback 1996
0-85198-986-1 £27.50

Bender, D.
An introduction to nutrition and metabolism
Taylor & Francis 368pp 2e. Paperback 1997
0-7484-0781-2 £21.99

Bender, D.A.
Nutrition: reference handbook
Oxford UP 612pp Paperback 1996
0-19-262368-0 £55.00

Garrow, J.S.
Human nutrition and dietetics
Churchill Liv 912pp 10e. Paperback 1999
0-443-05627-7 £48.95

Kopelman, P.G.
Clinical obesity
Blackwell Science UK 648pp Hardback 1998
0-632-04198-6 £75.00

Mahan, L.K.
Krause's food, nutrition, and diet therapy
W B Saunders 10e. 1344pp Paperback 1999
0-7216-7904-8 £46.95

Mann, J.
Essentials of human nutrition
Oxford UP 658pp Paperback 1998
0-19-262756-2 £29.95

Metcalfe, D.D.
Food allergy
Blackwell Science USA 800pp 2e. Hardback 1997
0-86542-432-2 £75.00

Payne-James, J.
Artificial nutrition support in clinical practice
Greenwich Medical 600pp 2e. Hardback 2000
1-900151-97-9 £100.00

Shaw, V.
Clinical paediatric dietetics
Blackwell Science Inc 480pp 2e. Paperback 2001
0632052414 £39.50

Shils, M.E.
Modern nutrition in health and disease
Williams and Wilkins 2100pp 9e. Hardback 1998
0-683-30769-X £75.00

Szmukler, G.
Handbook of eating disorders
John Wiley Ltd 438pp Paperback 1995
0-471-96307-0 £37.50

Thomas, B.
Manual of dietetic practice
Blackwell Science UK 752pp 2e. Paperback 1994
0-632-03003-8 £49.50

Truswell, S.
ABC of nutrition
BMJ Books 127pp Paperback 1999
0-7279-1233-X £16.95

Williams, S.R.
Essentials of nutrition and diet therapy
Mosby 657pp 7e. Paperback 1999
0-323-00398-2 £29.95

OBSTETRICS & GYNAECOLOGY

Bonnar, J.
Recent advances in obstetrics and gynaecology No. 20
Churchill Liv 234pp Paperback 1998
0-443-06022-3 £36.95

Campbell, S.
Gynaecology by ten teachers
Arnold 320pp 17e. Paperback 2000
0-340-71987-7 £17.99

Campbell, S.
Obstetrics by ten teachers
Arnold 320pp 17e. Paperback 2000
0-340-71986-9 £17.99

Cardozo, L.
Textbook of female urology and urogynecology
Isis Medical Media 800pp Hardback 2000
1-901865-05-3 £160.00

Chamberlain, G.
ABC of labour care
BMJ Books 58pp Paperback 1999
0-7279-1415-4 £12.95

Chamberlain, G.W.
Lecture notes on obstetrics and gynaecology
Blackwell Science UK 320pp 8e. Paperback 1999
0-632-04957-X £16.95

Chamberlain, G.
ABC of antenatal care
BMJ Books 100pp Paperback 1997
0-7279-1103-1 £15.95

Chamberlain, G.
Clinical physiology in obstetrics
Blackwell Science UK 480pp 3e. Hardback 1998
0-86542-948-0 £89.50

Chamberlain, G.
A practice of obstetrics and gynaecology
Churchill Liv 248pp 3e. Paperback 2000
0-443-05103-8 £29.95

Chamberlain, G.
Turnbull's obstetrics
Churchill Liv 914pp 2e. Hardback 1995
0-443-04998-X £132.00

Chard, T.
Basic sciences for obstetrics and gynaecology
Springer-Verlag 198pp 5e. Paperback 1997
3-540-76188-8 £19.50

Chudleigh, T.
Obstetric Ultrasound - How, Why and When
Churchill Liv 368pp 3e. Paperback 2000
0-443-05471-1 £29.50

Cox, C.
Managing obstetric emergencies
Bios Scientific 208pp Paperback 1999
1-85996-122-3 £19.95

Cunningham, F.G.
Williams obstetrics
Appleton and Lange 1472pp 20e. Paperback 1997
0-8385-9642-8 £70.00

DiSaia, P.J.
Clinical gynecologic oncology
Mosby 720pp 5e. Hardback 1997
0-8151-2506-2 £88.00

Dixon, J.M.
ABC of breast diseases
BMJ Books 96pp 2e. Paperback 2000
0-7279-1461-8 £16.95

Edmonds, K.
Dewhurst's textbook of obstetrics and gynaecology for postgraduates
Blackwell Science UK 832pp 6e. Hardback 1999
0-86542-651-1 £95.00

Enkin, M.
Guide to effective care in pregnancy and childbirth
Oxford UP Inc 432pp 3e. Paperback 2000
0-19-263173-X £14.99

Fentiman, I.S.
Detection and treatment of breast cancer
Martin Dunitz 300pp 2e. Hardback 1998
1-85317-223-5 £59.95

Gibb, D.
Fetal monitoring in practice
Butterworth-Heinemann 192pp 2e. Paperback 1997
0-7506-3432-4 £17.99

Greer, I.
Color atlas and text of obstetrics and gynecology
Mosby 352pp Paperback 2000
0-7234-2435-7 £26.95

Harris, J.R.
Diseases of the breast
Williams and Wilkins 2e. Hardback 2000
0-7817-1839-2 £124.00

Hillier, S.G.
Scientific essentials of reproductive medicine
W B Saunders Co Ltd 614pp Hardback 1996
0-7020-1826-0 £78.00

Hull, M.G.R.
Undergraduate obstetrics and gynaecology
Butterworth-Heinemann 473pp 3e. Paperback 1997
0-7506-1351-3 £22.50

Impey, L.
Obstetrics and gynaecology
Blackwell Science USA 320pp Paperback 1999
0-86542-704-6 £24.95

James, D.K.
High risk pregnancy
W B Saunders 1456pp 2e. Hardback 1999
0-7020-2223-3 £99.00

Johnson, M.H.
Essential reproduction
Blackwell Science 304pp 5e. Paperback 1999
0-632-04287-7 £24.95

Kaye, P.
Notes for the DRCOG
Churchill Liv 215pp 3e. Paperback 1995
0-443-04713-8 £23.95

Lewis, G.
Why mothers die: report on confidential enquiry into maternal deaths in the UK 1994-1996
Stationery Office 293pp Paperback 1998
0-11-322253-X £16.95

Llewellyn-Jones, D.
Fundamentals of obstetrics and gynaecology
W B Saunders 356pp 7e. Paperback 1999
0-7234-3150-7 £24.99

Loudon, N.
Handbook of family planning and reproductive healthcare
Churchill Liv 462pp 3e. Paperback 1995
0-443-05157-7 £43.95

McCarthy, A.
Obstetrics and gynaecology
Churchill Liv 264pp Paperback 1998
0-443-05244-1 £16.95

Meire, H.
Clinical ultrasound
Churchill Liv 736pp 2e. Hardback 2000
0-443-06154-8 £130.00

Miller, A.W.F.
Obstetrics illustrated
Churchill Liv 426pp 5e. Paperback 1997
0-443-05041-4 £26.95

Rock, J.A.
Te Linde's operative gynecology
Williams and Wilkins 1696pp 8e. Hardback 1997
0-397-51399-2 £108.50

Rubin, P.C.
Prescribing in pregnancy
BMJ Books 180pp 3e. Paperback 2000
0-7279-1449-9 £19.95

Russell, R.
Pain relief in labour
BMJ Books 256pp Paperback 1997
0-7279-1009-4 £27.00

Sharif, K.W.
MRCOG survival guide
W B Saunders 256pp 2e. Paperback 1999
0-7020-2545-3 £19.95

Shaw, R.W.
Gynaecology
Churchill Liv 961pp 2e. Hardback 1997
0-443-05231-X £126.00

Slade, R.
Key topics in obstetrics and gynaecology
Bios Scientific 336pp 2e. Paperback 1998
1-85996-226-2 £21.95

Stabile, I.
Clinical obstetrics and gynaecology
Springer-Verlag UK 250pp 2e. Paperback 2000
1-85233-615-3 £24.50

Studd, J.
Progress in obstetrics and gynaecology No. 13
Churchill Liv 432pp Paperback 1998
0-443-05868-7 £37.50

Swiet, M.de.
Medical disorders in obstetric practice
Blackwell Science UK 696pp 3e. Hardback 1995
0-632-03671-0   £69.50

Symonds, E.M.
Essential obstetrics and gynaecology
Churchill Liv 336pp Paperback 1997
0-443-05453-3   £24.95

Willocks, J.
Obstetrics and gynaecology
Churchill Liv 321pp 5e. Paperback 1997
0-443-04850-9   £19.95

OCCUPATIONAL THERAPY

Case-Smith, J.
Occupational therapy for children
Mosby 752pp Hardback 1996
0-8151-1541-5   £42.95

Case-Smith, J.
**Pediatric occupational therapy and early
intervention**
Butterworth-Heinemann 480pp 3e. Hardback 1998
0-7506-9780-6   £45.00

Cooper, J.
**Occupational therapy in oncology and palliative
care**
Whurr Publishers 310pp Paperback 1997
1-86156-015-X   £19.50

Creek, J.
Occupational therapy: new perspectives
Whurr Publishers 172pp Paperback 1998
1-86156-088-5   £19.50

Creek, J.
Occupational therapy and mental health
Churchill Liv 545pp 2e. Paperback 1996
0-443-05202-6   £34.95

Cynkin, S.
Occupational therapy and activities health
Williams and Wilkins 304pp Hardback 1989
0-316-16611-1   £33.50

Dimond, B.
Legal aspects of occupational therapy
Blackwell Science UK 400pp Paperback 1996
0-632-04074-2   £16.99

Grieve, J.
Neuropsychology for occupational therapists
Blackwell Science UK Paperback 1999
0-632-05067-5   £17.99

Hagedorn, R.
Foundations for practice in occupational therapy
Churchill Liv 157pp 2e. Paperback 1996
0-443-05292-1   £18.95

Hagedorn, R.
Occupational therapy
Churchill Liv 328pp 2e. Paperback 1995
0-443-04978-5   £21.95

Hansen, R.
Conditions in occupational therapy
Williams and Wilkins 2e. Paperback 1999
0-683-30417-8   £25.00

Jacobs, K.
**Quick reference dictionary for occupational
therapy**
Slack Inc 336pp Paperback 1999
1-55642-412-4   £16.50

Kielhofner, G.
Conceptual foundations of occupational therapy
F A Davis 350pp 2e. Hardback 1997
0-8036-0256-1   £37.95

Kielhofner, G.
A model of human occupation
Williams and Wilkins 501pp 2e. Paperback 1995
0-683-04601-2   £29.95

Kramer, P.
**Frames of reference for pediatric occupational
therapy**
Williams and Wilkins 2e. 625pp Hardback 1999
0-683-30489-5   £33.00

Law, M.C.
Client centered occupational therapy
Slack Inc 200pp Paperback 1998
1-55642-264-4   £22.50

Logigian, K.
Functions of a manager in occupational therapy
Slack Inc 200pp 3e. Paperback 1999
1-55642-374-8   £22.50

Martin, J.E.
Eating disorders, food and occupational therapy
Whurr Publishers 200pp Paperback 1998
1-86156-105-9   £19.50

Maslin, Z.
Management in occupational therapy
Stanley Thornes 240pp Paperback 1990
1-412-33380-5   £19.50

Miller, R.
**Perspectives on theory and practice in
occupational therapy**
Aspen Publishers 320pp 2e. Hardback 1993
0-8342-0358-8   £37.00

Mosey, A.C.
Psychosocial components of occupational therapy
Williams and Wilkins 624pp Hardback 1997
0-89004-334-5 £37.00

Neistadt, M.E.
Willard and Spackman's occupational therapy
Williams and Wilkins 960pp 9e. Hardback 1998
0-397-55192-4 £35.00

Pedretti, L.W.
Occupational therapy
Mosby 928pp 4e. Hardback 1996
0-8151-6812-8 £42.95

Punwar, A.
Occupational therapy: principles and practice
Lippincott Williams & Wilkins 304pp 3e.
Paperback 2000
0-683-30453-4 £23.95

Reed, K.
Concepts of occupational therapy
Williams and Wilkins 530pp 4e. Hardback 1999
0-683-30454-2 £28.50

Reed, K.
Quick reference to occupational therapy
Aspen Publishers 2e. 1006pp Paperback 2000
0-8342-1631-0 £36.00

Stein, F.
Psychosocial occupational therapy
Singular 300pp Paperback 1998
1-56593-925-5 £35.00

Sumsion, T.
Client centred practice in occupational therapy
Churchill Liv 144pp Paperback 1999
0-443-06127-0 £15.95

Trombly, C.A.
Occupational therapy for physical dysfunction
Williams and Wilkins 704pp 4e. Hardback 1995
0-683-08390-2 £29.95

Turner, A.
Occupational therapy and physical dysfunction
Churchill Liv 912pp 4e. Paperback 1996
0-443-05177-1 £43.95

Willson, M.
Occupational therapy in short-term psychiatry
Churchill Liv 269pp 3e. Paperback 1996
0-443-05396-0 £19.95

Wilson, E.
Occupational therapy for children with special needs
Whurr Publishers 250pp Paperback 1998
1-86156-061-3 £19.50

ONCOLOGY & RADIOTHERAPY
(See also Obstetrics & Gynecology, Palliative Care)

Abeloff, M.D.
Clinical oncology
Churchill Liv 2376pp 2e. 1999
0-443-07545-X Hardback £150.00
0-443-07555-7 CD-ROM £231.48

Allen-Mersh, T.G.
Surgical oncology
Arnold 480pp 6e. 1995
0-412-48940-6 Hardback £95.00
0-412-48950-3 Paperback £35.00

Andrassy, R.J.
Pediatric surgical oncology
W B Saunders 520pp Hardback 1998
0-7216-6378-8 £119.00

Bishop, J.F.
Cancer facts
Harwood Academic 422pp 1999
0-5702-365-2 Hardback £48.00
0-5702-470-5 Paperback £25.00

Cavalli, F.
Textbook of medical oncology
Martin Dunitz 800pp 2e. Hardback 1999
1-85317-825-X £99.50

De Vita, V.T.
Cancer: principles and practice of oncology
Lippincott Williams & Wilkins 3456pp 6e.
Hardback 2000
0-7817-2229-2 £164.00

Dobbs, J.
Practical radiotherapy planning
Arnold 350pp 3e. Paperback 1999
0-340-70631-7 £32.50

Feig, B.W.
The M.D. Anderson surgical oncology handbook
Williams and Wilkins 496pp 2e. Paperback 1998
0-7817-1581-4 £26.00

Harnett, P.
Oncology: a case-based manual
Oxford UP 212pp Paperback 1999
0-19-262978-6 £19.95

Kurzrock, R.
Molecular biology in cancer medicine
Martin Dunitz 600pp 2e. Hardback 1999
1-85317-676-1 £75.00

Leibel, S.A.
Textbook of radiation oncology
W B Saunders 1376pp Hardback 1998
0-7216-5336-7 £159.00

McKinnell, R.G.
The biological basis of cancer
Cambridge UP 398pp 1998
0-521-59298-4 Hardback £70.00
0-521-59695-5 Paperback £27.95

Neal, A.J.
Clinical oncology
Arnold 256pp 2e. Paperback 1997
0-340-67748-1 £17.99

Peckham, M.
Oxford textbook of oncology
Oxford UP 1200pp Hardback 1995
0-19-261685-4 £245.00

Pollock, R.E.
Manual of clinical oncology
John Wiley Inc 826pp 7e. Hardback 1999
0-471-23828-7 £45.50

Roses, D.F.
Breast cancer - physician volume
Churchill Liv 704pp Hardback 1999
0-443-05581-5 £110.00

Skeel, R.T.
Handbook of cancer chemotherapy
Williams and Wilkins 608pp 5e. Paperback 1999
0-7817-1617-9 £28.00

Souhami, R.L.
Cancer and its management
Blackwell Science USA 536pp 3e. Hardback 1998
0-86542-774-7 £29.95

Tannock, I.F.
The basic science of oncology
McGraw-Hill HPD 430pp 3e. Paperback 1998
0-07-105484-7 £39.99

Tobias, J.S.
Breast cancer: new horizons in research and treatment
Arnold 368pp Hardback 2000
0-340-74216-X £85.00

Tobias, J.S.
Current radiation oncology - 3
Arnold 424pp Hardback 1997
0-340-67739-2 £69.00

Twycross, R.
Symptom management in advanced cancer
Radcliffe Medical 384pp 2e. Paperback 1997
1-85775-282-1 £24.95

Voute, P.A.
Cancer in children
Oxford UP 372pp 4e. Hardback 1998
0-19-262897-6 £49.95

OPHTHALMOLOGY

Adams, G.
Kennerley Bankes's clinical ophthalmology
Butterworth-Heinemann 200pp 4e. Paperback 1999
0-7506-3908-3 £22.50

Bartlett, J.D.
Clinical ocular pharmacology
Butterworth-Heinemann 1120pp 4e. Hardback 2000
0-7506-7039-8 £95.00

Batterbury, M.
Ophthalmology
Churchill Liv 128pp Paperback 1999
0-443-05537-8 £16.95

Bron, A.
Ocular infection
Martin Dunitz 180pp Paperback 1998
1-85317-437-8 £35.00

Bron, A.J.
Lens disorders
Butterworth-Heinemann 256pp Hardback 1995
0-7506-1482-X £85.00

Chawla, H.B.
Ophthalmology: a symptom-based approach
Butterworth-Heinemann 256pp 3e. Paperback 1999
0-7506-3979-2 £25.00

Chawla, H.B.
Retinal detachment
Butterworth-Heinemann 160pp 3e. Paperback 1998
0-7506-3980-6 £35.00

Crick, R.P.
Textbook of clinical ophthalmology
World Scientific 616pp 2e. Paperback 1997
981-02-2373-0 £35.00

Easty, D.
Oxford textbook of ophthalmology
Oxford UP 1396pp Hardback 1999
0-19-262557-8 £225.00

Evans, N.
Ophthalmology
Oxford UP 296pp 1995
0-19-262407-5 Hardback £55.00
0-19-262406-7 Paperback £27.50

Forrester, J.V.
The eye: basic sciences in practice
W B Saunders Co Ltd 424pp Paperback 1995
0-7020-1790-6 £53.00

Foss, A.
Essential ophthalmic surgery
Butterworth-Heinemann 448pp Paperback 2000
0-7506-4197-5 £35.00

Gasson, A.
Contact lens manual
Butterworth-Heinemann 352pp 2e. Paperback 1998
0-7506-3187-2 £37.50

Good, W.
Strabismus management
Butterworth-Heinemann 432pp Hardback 1995
0-7506-9075-5 £72.00

Hoh, B.
Clinical cases in ophthalmology
Butterworth-Heinemann 224pp Paperback 1995
0-7506-2102-8 £32.50

Hung Cheng
Emergency ophthalmology: a symptom based guide
BMJ Books 344pp Paperback 1997
0-7279-0861-8 £50.00

James, B.
Lecture notes on ophthalmology
Blackwell Science UK 208pp 8e. Paperback 1996
0-86542-723-2 £14.95

Kanski, J.J.
Clinical ophthalmology
Butterworth-Heinemann 560pp 4e. Hardback 1999
0-7506-4014-6 £105.00

Kanski, J.J.
Glaucoma
Butterworth-Heinemann 192pp 2e. Hardback 1995
0-7506-1820-5 £65.00

Khaw, P.T.
ABC of eyes
BMJ Books 61pp 3e. Paperback 1999
0-7279-1262-3 £16.95

Khaw, P.T.
Ophthalmology revision aid
BMJ Books 304pp 2e. Paperback 1996
0-7279-1011-6 £25.00

Newell, F.W.
Ophthalmology: principles and concepts
Mosby 608pp 8e. Hardback 1996
0-8151-7093-9 £59.00

Phillips, A.J.
Contact lenses
Butterworth-Heinemann 889pp 4e. Mixed-media pack 1997
0-7506-1819-1 £80.00

Rhee, D.J.
The Wills eye manual
Williams and Wilkins 480pp 3e. Paperback 1999
0-7817-1602-0 £35.00

Rowe, F.J.
Clinical orthoptics
Blackwell Science UK 288pp Paperback 1997
0-632-04274-5 £29.50

Roy, F.H.
Ocular differential diagnosis
Williams and Wilkins 700pp 6e. Paperback 1996
0-683-07415-6 £52.00

Snell, R.S.
Clinical anatomy of the eye
Blackwell Science USA 368pp 2e. Paperback 1998
0-632-04344-X £39.50

Spalton, D.J.
Atlas of clinical ophthalmology
Mosby 568pp 2e. Hardback 1993
0-397-44632-2 £135.00

Taylor, D.
Practical paediatric ophthalmology
Blackwell Science UK 283pp Paperback 1996
0-86542-720-8 £34.50

Towler, H.
Diabetes and the eye CD-ROM
BMJ Books 2e. 1998
0-7279-1381-6 £99.88

Vaughan, D.
General ophthalmology
Appleton and Lange 350pp 15e. Paperback 1998
0-8385-3137-7 £31.00

Webb, L.
Eye emergencies
Butterworth-Heinemann 196pp Paperback 1995
0-7506-2015-3 £21.50

Yanoff, M.
Ocular pathology
Mosby 744pp 4e. 1995
0-7234-2199-4 Hardback £159.00
0-7234-2229-X CD-ROM £182.13

ORTHOPAEDICS
(See also Physiotherapy, Podiatry)

Adams, J.C.
Outline of orthopaedics
Churchill Liv 448pp 12e. Hardback 1995
0-443-05149-6 £23.95

Adams, J.C.
Outline of fractures.
Churchill Liv 328pp 11e. Paperback 1999
0-443-06027-4 £22.00

Adams, J.C.
Standard orthopaedic operations
Churchill Liv 485pp 4e. Hardback 1992
0-443-04351-5 £126.00

Andrew, J.E.
Musculoskeletal medicine and surgery
Churchill Liv 368pp Paperback 2000
0-443-05698-6 £19.95

Apley, A.G.
Concise system of orthopaedics and fractures
Butterworth-Heinemann 336pp 2e. Paperback 1994
0-7506-1767-5 £16.99

Broughton, N.
Paediatric orthopaedics
W B Saunders Co Ltd 384pp Hardback 1996
0-7020-1962-3 £62.00

Canale, S.T.
Campbell's operative orthopedics
4 vols Mosby 4704pp 1998
0-8151-2087-7 Hardback £315.00
0-323-00494-6 CD-ROM £312.55

Cyriax, J.H.
Cyriax's illustrated manual of orthopaedic medicine
Butterworth-Heinemann 279pp 2e. Paperback 1996
0-7506-3274-7 £40.00

Dandy, D.J.
Essential orthopaedics and trauma
Churchill Liv 488pp 3e. Paperback 1998
0-443-05724-9 £23.95

Duckworth, T.
Lecture notes on orthopaedics and fractures
Blackwell Science UK 447pp 3e. Paperback 1995
0-632-02781-9 £16.95

Duthie, R.B.
Mercer's orthopaedic surgery
Arnold 1376pp 9e. Hardback 1996
0-340-55163-1 £150.00

Goldie, B.
Orthopaedic diagnosis and management
Isis Medical Media 368pp 2e. Paperback 1998
1-899066-90-X £24.95

Huckstep, R.L.
A simple guide to trauma
Churchill Liv 515pp 5e. Paperback 1995
0-443-04679-4 £12.95

Hughes, S.P.F.
Textbook of orthopaedics and fractures
Arnold 256pp Paperback 1997
0-340-61381-5 £18.99

Jones, A.E.
Color atlas of clinical orthopaedics
Mosby 256pp 2e. Hardback 1994
0-7234-2058-0 £82.00

Keene, G.S.
Key topics in orthopaedic trauma surgery
Bios Scientific 320pp Paperback 1999
1-85996-291-2 £23.95

Macnicol, M.
The problem knee
Butterworth-Heinemann 224pp 2e. Paperback 1998
0-7506-4044-8 £27.50

McRae, R.
Clinical orthopaedic examination
Churchill Liv 308pp 4e. Paperback 1997
0-443-05602-1 £22.95

McRae, R.
Practical fracture treatment
Churchill Liv 389pp 3e. Paperback 1994
0-443-04809-6 £31.95

Rockwood Jr, C.A.
Fractures in children
Williams and Wilkins 1552pp Hardback 1996
0-397-51512-X £132.00

Rockwood Jr, C.A.
Fractures in adults
2 vols Williams and Wilkins 1552pp Hardback 1996
0-397-51602-9 £227.00

Rockwood Jr, C.A.
Fractures
Williams and Wilkins 1552pp Hardback 1996
0-397-51775-0 CD-ROM £340.75

Solomon, L.
Physical examination in orthopaedics
Butterworth-Heinemann 113pp Paperback 1995
0-7506-1766-7 £16.50

Solomon, L.
Apley's system of orthopaedics and fractures
Butterworth-Heinemann 608pp 8e. Hardback 2000
0-7506-4156-8 £89.50

Weinstein, S.L.
Turek's orthopaedics
Williams and Wilkins 832pp 5e. Hardback 1994
0-397-50692-9 £103.50

PAEDIATRICS

Advanced Life Support Group
Advanced paediatric life support
BMJ Books 320pp 2e. Paperback 1997
0-7279-1069-8 £25.00

Appleton, R.E.
Epilepsy in childhood and adolescence pocketbook
Martin Dunitz 120pp 2e. Paperback 1998
1-85317-654-0 £14.95

Archer, N.
Paediatric cardiology
Arnold 240pp Hardback 1998
0-412-73450-8 £45.00

Armstrong, H.
A safer practice: child protection guide
Stationery Office 18pp Paperback 1996
0-11-321991-1 £19.95

Attard-Montalto, S.
Paediatrics
Churchill Liv 272pp Paperback 1999
0-443-05516-5 £15.95

Behrman, R.E.
Nelson essentials of pediatrics
W B Saunders 846pp 3e. Paperback 1998
0-7216-7229-9 £35.00

Behrman, R.E.
Nelson textbook of pediatrics
W B Saunders 2480pp 16e. Hardback 1999
0-7216-7767-3 £75.00

Bellman, M.H.
Paediatrics and Child Health: A Textbook for the DCH
Churchill Liv 404pp Paperback 2000
0-443-05901-2 £36.95

Brett, E.M.
Paediatric neurology
Churchill Liv 928pp 3e. Hardback 1997
0-443-05200-X £158.00

British Medical Association
Growing up in Britain
BMA Professional 221pp Paperback 1999
0-7279-1433-2 £19.95

Brook, C.G.D.
Clinical paediatric endocrinology
Blackwell Science UK 832pp 3e. Hardback 1995
0-632-03632-X £149.50

Buckler, J.F.M.D.D.
A reference manual of growth and development
Blackwell Science UK 128pp 2e. Paperback 1997
0-86542-680-5 £16.95

Cade, A.
Short cases for the paediatric MRCP
Greenwich Medical 208pp Paperback 2000
1-84110-009-9 £22.50

Campbell, A.G.M.
Forfar and Arneil's textbook of pediatrics
Churchill Liv 2080pp 5e. Hardback 1997
0-443-05393-6 £155.00

David, T.J.
Recent advances in paediatrics-18
Churchill Liv 264pp Paperback 2000
0-443-06430-X £35.00

David, T.J.
Symptoms of disease in childhood
Blackwell Science UK 292pp Paperback 1995
0-632-03635-4 £15.95

Davies, E.G.
Manual of childhood infections
W B Saunders 2e. Paperback 1999
0-7020-2379-5 £18.95

Dubowitz, V.
Muscle disorders in childhood
W B Saunders Co Ltd 460pp 2e. Hardback 1995
0-7020-1437-0 £83.00

Fleisher, G.R.
Textbook of pediatric emergency medicine
Williams and Wilkins 2030pp 4e. Hardback 1999
0-683-30609-X £125.00

Gill, D.
Paediatric clinical examination
Churchill Liv 264pp 3e. Paperback 1998
0-443-05961-6 £12.95

Glasgow, J.
Management of injuries in children
BMJ Books 300pp Paperback 1997
0-7279-0925-8 £38.00

Hall, D.
The child surveillance handbook
Radcliffe Medical 288pp 2e. Paperback 1999
1-870905-24-5 £19.95

Hall, D.M.B.
The child with a disability
Blackwell Science UK 400pp 2e. Paperback 1997
0-632-04776-3 £29.50

Hall, D.M.B.
Health for all children
Oxford UP 268pp 3e. Paperback 1996
0-19-262656-6 £12.99

Hann, I.M.
Colour atlas of paediatric haematology
Oxford UP 202pp 3e. Hardback 1996
0-19-262696-5 £99.50

Hull, D.
Essential paediatrics
Churchill Liv 400pp 4e. Paperback 1999
0-443-05958-6 £24.95

Hutson, J.M.
Jones' clinical paediatric surgery
Blackwell Science 320pp 5e. Paperback 1999
0-86793-012-8   £35.00

Insley, J.
A paediatric vade-mecum
Arnold 448pp 13e. Paperback 1996
0-340-60158-2   £16.99

Johnston, P.G.B.
The newborn child
Churchill Liv 268pp Paperback 1998
0-443-05510-6   £19.95

Jones, D.
Child sexual abuse
Radcliffe Medical 120pp Paperback 1999
1-85775-362-3   £14.95

Jones, K.L.
Smith's recognizable patterns of human malformation
W B Saunders 880pp Hardback 1997
0-7216-6115-7   £55.00

Jones, P.F.
Emergency abdominal surgery in infancy
Hodder & Stoughton 3e. Hardback 1998
0-412-81950-3   £47.50

Kelnar, C.J.H.
The sick newborn baby
Bailliere Tindall 484pp 3e. Paperback 1995
0-7020-1647-0   £17.95

Klaus, M.H.
Care of the high-risk neonate
W B Saunders 5e. 555pp Hardback 2001
0-7216-7729-0   £40.00

Levene, M.
Essentials of neonatal medicine
Blackwell Science UK 352pp 3e. Paperback 2000
0-632-05163-9   £24.95

Levene, M.
Paediatrics and child health
Blackwell Science UK 416pp Paperback 1999
0-86542-957-X   £24.95

Lilleyman, J.S.
Pediatric hematology
Churchill Liv 944pp 2e. Hardback 1999
0-443-05840-7   £125.00

Lissauer, T.
Illustrated textbook of paediatrics
Mosby 352pp Paperback 1996
0-7234-1657-5   £25.95

Meadow, R.
ABC of child abuse
BMJ Books 96pp 3e. Paperback 1997
0-7279-1106-6   £16.95

Milner, A.D.
Hospital paediatrics
Churchill Liv 440pp 3e. Paperback 1997
0-443-05392-8   £31.95

Mowat, A.P.
Liver disorders in childhood
Butterworth-Heinemann 496pp 3e. Paperback 1994
0-7506-4200-9   £55.00

Moyer, V.A.
Evidence based paediatrics and child health
BMJ Books 700pp Hardback 2000
0-7279-1424-3   £85.00

Phelan, P.D.
Respiratory illness in children
Blackwell Science UK 448pp 4e. Paperback 1994
0-632-03764-4   £65.00

Polnay, L.
Manual of community paediatrics
Churchill Liv 309pp 2e. Paperback 1996
0-443-05352-9   £21.95

Roberton, N.R.C.
A manual of neonatal intensive care
Arnold 496pp 4e. Paperback 2000
0-340-72010-7   £17.99

Roberton, N.R.C.
Textbook of neonatology
Churchill Liv 1504pp 3e. Hardback 1999
0-443-05541-6   £185.00

Robinson, M.J.
Practical paediatrics
Churchill Liv 824pp 4e. Paperback 1998
0-443-05893-8   £42.00

Sinclair, D.
Human growth after birth
Oxford UP 264pp 6e. Paperback 1998
0-19-262905-0   £18.95

Stephenson, T.
Clinical paediatrics for postgraduate examinations
Churchill Liv 212pp 2e. Paperback 1995
0-443-05226-3   £23.95

Taeusch, H.W.
Averys' diseases of the newborn
W B Saunders 1360pp 7e. Hardback 1998
0-7216-5751-6   £99.00

Taylor, S.
Diagnosis in color: pediatrics
Mosby 384pp Paperback 1997
0-7234-2494-2   £21.95

Valman, B.
ABC of one to seven
Books 160pp 4e. Paperback 1999
0-7279-1232-1   £17.95

Valman, H.B.
The first year of life
BMJ Books 112pp 4e. Paperback 1995
0-7279-0897-9   £13.95

Walker-Smith, J.
Diseases of the small intestine in childhood
Isis Medical Media 424pp Hardback 1999
1-901865-03-7   £99.50

Waterston, T.
Paediatrics
Oxford UP 432pp 1997
0-19-262564-0 Hardback   £45.00
0-19-262563-2 Paperback   £19.95

Wright, K.W.
Pediatric ophthalmology for pediatricians
Williams and Wilkins Paperback 364pp
0-683-30485-2   £41.00

PALLIATIVE & TERMINAL CARE

Clark, D.
New themes in palliative care
Open UP 224pp Paperback 1997
0-335-19605-5   £22.50

Clark, D.
Reflections on palliative care
Open UP 219pp Paperback 1998
0-335-19454-0   £16.99

Cooper, J.
Stepping into palliative care
Radcliffe Medical 264pp Paperback 2000
1-85775-303-8   £17.95

Doyle, D.
Oxford textbook of palliative medicine
Oxford UP 1308pp 2e. 1997
0-19-262566-7 Hardback   £79.50
0-19-263057-1 Paperback   £49.95

Dunlop, R.
Cancer: palliative care
Springer-Verlag Berl 181pp Paperback 1997
3-540-19974-8   £19.95

Faull, C.
The handbook of palliative care
Blackwell Science UK 300pp Paperback 1998
0-632-04779-8   £27.50

Goldman, A.
Care of the dying child
Oxford UP 224pp Paperback 1994
0-19-261983-7   £24.95

Hindmarch, C.
On the death of a child
Radcliffe Medical 136pp Paperback 2000
1-85775-445-X   £14.95

MacDonald, N.
Palliative medicine
Oxford UP 330pp Paperback 1997
0-19-262657-4   £16.95

Neuberger, J.
Caring for dying people of different faiths
Mosby 69pp Paperback 1994
0-7234-2154-4   £9.00

Parkes, C.M.
Coping with loss
BMJ Books 168pp Paperback 1998
0-7279-1068-X   £14.95

Parkes, C.M.
Counselling in terminal care and bereavement
Br Psychological Soc 215pp Paperback 1996
1-85433-178-7   £12.95

Penson, J.
Palliative care for people with cancer
Arnold 360pp 2e. Paperback 1995
0-340-61391-2   £16.99

Robbins, J.
Caring for the dying patient and the family
Stanley Thornes 298pp 3e. Paperback 1995
0-412-57840-9   £22.50

Robbins, M.
Evaluating palliative care
Oxford UP 186pp Paperback 1998
0-19-262621-3   £27.50

Saunders, C.
Living with dying
Oxford UP 76pp 3e. Paperback 1995
0-19-262514-4   £14.95

Twycross, R.
Introducing palliative care
Radcliffe Medical 200pp 3e. Paperback 1999
1-85775-389-5   £18.95

PATHOLOGY & LABORATORY MEDICINE

Burkitt, H.G.
Wheater's basic histopathology
Churchill Liv 288pp 3e. Paperback 1996
0-443-05088-0   £35.95

Burtis, C.A.
Tietz fundamentals of clinical chemistry
W B Saunders 912pp 4e. Hardback 1995
0-7216-3763-9   £47.95

Burtis, C.A.
Tietz textbook of clinical chemistry
W B Saunders 2000pp 3e. Hardback 1998
0-7216-5610-2   £135.00

Cook, D.J.
Cellular pathology
Butterworth-Heinemann 383pp Paperback 1998
0-7506-3111-2   £19.99

Cotran, R.S.
Robbins pathologic basis of disease
W B Saunders 1472pp 6e. Hardback 1998
0-7216-7335-X   £52.95

Cree, I.A.
Pathology
Arnold 608pp Paperback 1997
0-412-47200-7   £32.95

Crocker, J.
The science of laboratory diagnosis
Isis Medical Media 600pp Paperback 1998
1-899066-62-4   £59.95

Curran, R.
Curran's histopathology
Oxford UP 304pp 4e. Paperback 2000
0-19-263220-5   £24.50

Damjanov, I.
Anderson's pathology
2 vols Mosby 3030pp 10e. Hardback 1996
0-8016-7236-8   £235.00

Damjanov, I.
Pathology: a color atlas
Mosby 544pp Hardback 1999
0-8151-2248-9   £130.00

Henry, J.B.
Clinical diagnosis and management by laboratory methods
W B Saunders 19e. 1580pp Hardback 1996
0-7216-6030-4   £69.00

Jones, R.
Clinical investigation and statistics in laboratory medicine
ACB Venture Pub 188pp Paperback 1997
0-902429-21-3   £21.00

Kumar, V.
Basic pathology
W B Saunders 784pp 6e. Hardback 1997
0-7216-5122-4   £37.95

Macfarlane, P.
Pathology illustrated
Churchill Liv 696pp 5e. Paperback 1999
0-443-05956-X   £34.95

MacSween, R.N.M.
Muir's textbook of pathology
Arnold 14e. Paperback 2000
0-340-74062-0   £35.00

Marshall, W.J.
Clinical biochemistry
Mosby 854pp Paperback 1995
0-443-04341-8   £110.00

Marshall, W.J.
Clinical chemistry
Mosby 336pp Paperback 2000
0-7234-3159-0   £21.95

Mayne, P.D.
Clinical chemistry in diagnosis and treatment
Arnold 480pp 6e. Paperback 1994
0-340-57647-2   £16.99

Mitchinson, M.J.
Essentials of pathology
Blackwell Science UK 352pp Paperback 1995
0-632-02944-7   £15.95

Pallister, C.
Baker and Silverton's introduction to medical laboratory technology
Butterworth-Heinemann 432pp 7e. Paperback 1998
0-7506-2190-7   £37.50

Parums, D.V.
Essential clinical pathology
Blackwell Science UK 736pp Paperback 1996
0-632-03088-7   £29.95

Rosai, J.
Ackerman's surgical pathology
Mosby 2796pp 8e. 1995
0-8016-7004-7 Hardback   £250.00
0-8151-3773-7 CD-ROM   £276.13

Rubin, E.
Essential pathology
Williams and Wilkins 832pp 2e. Hardback 1995
0-397-51487-5   £29.50

Rubin, E.
Pathology
Williams and Wilkins 1648pp 3e. Hardback 1998
0-397-58422-9   £37.00

Smith, A.F.
Lecture notes on clinical biochemistry
Blackwell Science UK 328pp 6e. Paperback 1998
0-632-04834-4   £16.95

New & Classic Ophthalmology Titles

Clinical Ophthalmology 4e
Jack J Kanski
This classic text, with its broad coverage, systematic presentation and numerous superb full colour illustrations is a world-wide bestseller having been translated into 8 languages. It remains an essential text for the trainee ophthalmologist.
1999   0750640146   £110.00   696pp   9x216mm

...hepens' Retinal Detachment and Allied ...seases 2e
...arles L Schepens
...w published by BH, this up-to-date and authoritative clinical ...erence provides you with everything you need to know ...out retinal detachment. This highly-illustrated book not only ...vers the advances in surgical procedures but also empha-...es differential diagnosis and follow-up. Ophthalmologists ...l benefit from the author's years of experience in treating ...inal disorders.
...ne 2000   0750698373   £240.00   784pp   279x216mm

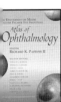

The University of Miami Bascom Palmer Eye Institute Atlas of Ophthalmology
Richard K Parrish II (Ed.)
A full-color atlas covering all areas of ophthalmology from one of the premier eye centers in the world. This unique atlas, available in both print form and on CD-ROM (Win 3.1+, Mac System 7+), is a comprehensive four-color atlas that will aid the diagnosis and treatment of ophthalmic conditions.
...99   0750670754   £150.00   678pp   279x216mm
...-ROM: 2000   0750670762   £140.00 + vat

...trabismus 4e
...lio Prieto-Diaz & Carlos Souza-Dias
...his textbook is already a classic in Latin America and now ...translation into English makes it available to an even wider ...dience. The authority of this textbook is apparent on every ...ge. The authors are experienced practitioners who have ...so thought long and hard about the tough problems in stra-...smus theory and practice. The illustrations are plentiful and ...ear. The references reveal the wide range of these authors' ...holarship. This is a book that can be used as a textbook to ...e read from cover to cover or to explore selected topics." - ...om the Foreword by Creig S. Hoyt, MD (University of ...alifornia, San Francisco)
...00   0750671297   £110.00   608pp   279x216pp

Kennerley Bankes`s Clinical Ophthalmology 4e
Gillian Adams & Alan Hubbard
Completely updated and revised, and under new authorship, this text with its superb full colour illustrations and concise text provides a valuable introduction to clinical ophthalmology for medical students, general medical practitioners and all those involved in clinical eye care.
1999   0750639083   £23.50   200pp   246x189mm

Ophthalmology: a Symptom Based Approach 3e
Hector Bryson Chawla
A witty and painless introduction to ophthalmology, this revised third edition of Dr Chawla's popular book provides medical students with the essential core of knowledge necessary for examinations. The book will be invaluable to trainee ophthalmologists, optometrists, ophthalmic nurses and general practitioners.
1999   0750639792   £25.99   224pp   246x189mm

The Pupil
Irene E Loewenfeld
This two-volume reference offers a comprehensive synthesis of all the information available on the pupil from many disciplines, including anatomy, physiology, pharmacology, neurology, ophthalmology, and internal medicine.
1999   0750671432   £180.00   2223pp   279x216mm

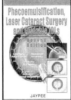

Phacoemulsification, Laser Cataract Surgery andFodlable IOLs 2/e
Sunita Agarwal et al
A book that presents the most advanced techniques of cataract surgery. This new edition has been enlarged and updated with the latest information in the field. Highly illustrated.
2000 8171797601 £80.00 626pp 285x217mm

Ocular Tumours
Bertil Damato
Thoroughly referenced, this text contains the theory as well as adopting a practical approach. The approach is systematic and detailed, covering all aspects of ocular tumours, including clinical features, diagnosis and management.
Superbly illustrated with high quality colour photographs.
2000   0750622202   £75.00   288pp   246x189mm

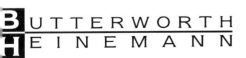

BUTTERWORTH HEINEMANN

http://www.bh.com
For more information please contact Catherine Jackson
Linacre House, Jordan Hill, Oxford, OX2 8DP
Fax 01865 314519 email catherine.jackson@repp.co.uk

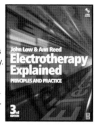

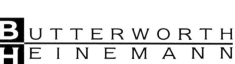
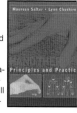

Spector, T.D.
Introduction to general pathology
Churchill Liv 404pp 4e. Paperback 1999
0-443-04884-3 £17.50

Stevens, A.
Pathology
Mosby 664pp 2e. Paperback 2000
0-7234-3160-4 £33.95

Tomlinson, S.
Mechanisms of disease
Cambridge UP 531pp 1997
0-521-46180-4 Hardback £60.00
0-521-46738-1 Paperback £20.95

Underwood, J.C.E.
General and systematic pathology
Churchill Liv 848pp 3e. Paperback 2000
0-443-06285-4 £37.95

Walmsley, R.N.
A guide to diagnostic clinical chemistry
Blackwell Science UK 672pp 3e. Hardback 1996
0-632-03735-0 £52.50

Walter, J.B.
General pathology
Churchill Liv 952pp 7e. Hardback 1995
0-443-04296-9 £99.95

PHARMACOLOGY & TOXICOLOGY

American Academy of Pediatrics
Handbook of common poisonings in children
American Acad Pediat 280pp Paperback 1998
0-910761-58-2 £35.00

Bates, N.
Paediatric toxicology: handbook of poisoning in children
Macmillan Reference 424pp Hardback 1997
0-333-60951-4 £59.00

British Medical Association
BMA new guide to medicines & drugs
Dorling Kindersley 480pp Hardback 2000
0-7513-0444-1 £14.99

Brody, T.M.
Human pharmacology
Mosby 1024pp 3e. Paperback 1998
0-8151-2456-2 £24.95

Department of Health
British pharmacopoeia: 2000
Stationery Office 3200pp Hardback 2000
0-11-322320-X £750.00

Foster, R.W.
Basic pharmacology
Butterworth-Heinemann 580pp 4e. Paperback 1996
0-7506-2198-2 £21.50

Greenwood, D.
Antimicrobial chemotherapy
Oxford UP 400pp 4e. Paperback 2000
0-19-263195-0 £29.95

Haddad, L.M.
Clinical management of poisoning and drug overdose
W B Saunders 1260pp 3e. Hardback 1997
0-7216-6409-1 £110.00

Hardman, J.G.
Goodman and Gilman's the pharmacological basis of therapeutics
McGraw-Hill HPD 9e. 1840pp 1996
0-07-026266-7 Hardback £72.99
0-07-864186-1 CD-ROM £78.00

Harvey, R.
Lippincotts' illustrated reviews: pharmacology
Williams and Wilkins 2e. Paperback 2000
0-7817-2413-9 £21.00

Katzung, B.G.
Basic and clinical pharmacology
Appleton and Lange 1000pp 7e. Paperback 1997
0-8385-0565-1 £29.99

Klaassen, C.D.
Casarett and Doull's toxicology
McGraw-Hill HPD 912pp Hardback 1996
0-07-105476-6 £52.99

Klaassen, C.D.
Casarett and Doull's toxicology: companion handbook
McGraw-Hill HPD 912pp 5e.Hardback 1996
0-07-034963-0 £25.00

Lambert, H.P.
Antibiotic and chemotherapy
Churchill Liv 987pp 7e. Hardback 1997
0-443-05255-7 £104.00

Laurence, D.R.
Clinical pharmacology
Churchill Liv 710pp 8e. Paperback 1997
0-443-04990-4 £38.95

Melmon, K.L.
Melmon and Morrelli's the essentials of clinical pharmacology
McGraw-Hill HPD 1200pp 4e. Paperback 2000
0-07-105406-5 £42.99

Olson, K.R.
Poisoning and drug overdose
Appleton and Lange 608pp 3e. Paperback 1998
0-8385-0260-1 £25.00

Page, C.
Integrated pharmacology
Mosby 618pp Paperback 1997
0-7234-2556-6   £35.95

Parfitt, K.
Martindale: extra pharmacopoeia
Pharmaceutical Press 2500pp 32e. Hardback 1999
0-85369-429-X   £235.00

Rang, H.P.
Pharmacology
Churchill Liv 832pp 4e. Paperback 1999
0-443-05974-8   £35.95

Reid, J.L.
Lecture notes on clinical pharmacology
Blackwell Science UK 432pp 5e. Paperback 1996
0-86542-665-1   £14.95

Ritter, J.M.
A textbook of clinical pharmacology
Arnold 704pp 4e. Paperback 1999
0-340-70593-0   £32.99

Speight, T.M.
Avery's drug treatment
Blackwell Science UK 1820pp 4e. Hardback 1997
0-86471-036-4   £90.00

Stockley, I.H.
Drug interactions
Pharmaceutical Press 1200pp 5e. Hardback 1999
0-85369-424-9   £69.00

Timbrell, J.
Principles of biochemical toxicology
Taylor & Francis 408pp 3e. Paperback 1999
0-7484-0736-7   £24.99

PHYSIOLOGY

Berne, R.A.
Physiology
Mosby 1110pp 4e. Hardback 1998
0-8151-0952-0   £33.95

Berne, R.M.
Principles of physiology
Mosby 800pp 3e. Paperback 2000
0-323-00813-5   £26.95

Bray, J.
Lecture notes on human physiology
Blackwell Science USA 672pp 4e. Paperback 1999
0-86542-775-5   £19.95

Despopoulos, A.
Color atlas of physiology
Thieme Verlag 379pp 4e. Paperback 1991
3-13-545004-X   £19.50

Fox, S.
Human physiology
Wm C Brown 688pp 5e. Hardback 1995
0-697-20985-7   £19.95

Ganong, W.F.
Review of medical physiology
Appleton and Lange 862pp 19e. Paperback 1999
0-8385-8252-4   £26.99

Guyton, A.C.
Human physiology and mechanisms of disease
W B Saunders 768pp 6e. Hardback 1996
0-7216-3299-8   £39.95

Guyton, A.C.
Textbook of medical physiology
W B Saunders 1075pp 10e. Hardback 2000
0-7216-8677-X   £33.95

MacKenna, B.R.
Illustrated physiology
Churchill Liv 336pp 6e. Paperback 1996
0-443-05060-0   £21.95

McGeown, G.
Physiology
Churchill Liv 236pp Paperback 1996
0-443-05196-8   £16.95

Pocock, G.
Human physiology
Oxford UP 646pp 1999
0-19-262539-X Hardback   £60.00
0-19-262538-1 Paperback   £27.50

Scratcherd, T.
Aids to physiology.
Churchill Liv 400pp 3e. Paperback 1997
0-443-05451-7   £19.95

Vander, A.J.
Human physiology
McGraw-Hill 768pp 8e. Paperback 2000
0-07-118254-3   £31.99

PHYSIOTHERAPY

Bookhout, M.R.
Bourdillon's spinal manipulation
Butterworth-Heinemann 375pp 6e. Hardback 2000
0-7506-7239-0   £47.50

Brimer, M.A.
Clinical cases in physical therapy
Butterworth-Heinemann 128pp Paperback 1995
0-7506-9637-0   £20.00

Bromley, I.
Tetraplegia and paraplegia
Churchill Liv 276pp 5e. Hardback 1998
0-443-05872-5   £29.95

Bury, T.
Evidence based healthcare: a practical guide for therapists
Butterworth-Heinemann 264pp Paperback 1998
0-7506-3783-8 £19.99

Buschbacher, R.
Musculoskeletal disorders: a practical guide for diagnosis and rehabilitation
Butterworth-Heinemann 326pp Hardback 1993
1-56372-077-9 £70.00

Campion, M.R.
Hydrotherapy: principles and practice
Butterworth-Heinemann Paperback 347pp 1996
0-7506-2261-X £29.50

Carr, J.H.
A motor relearning programme for stroke
Butterworth-Heinemann 208pp 2e. Paperback 1987
0-7506-0272-4 £40.00

Charman, R.A.
Complementary therapies for physiotherapists
Butterworth-Heinemann 320pp Paperback 2000
0-7506-4079-0 £29.99

David, C.
Rheumatological physiotherapy
Mosby 208pp Paperback 1998
0-7234-2594-9 £19.95

Dimond, B.C.
Legal aspects of physiotherapy
Blackwell Science UK 448pp Paperback 1999
0-632-05108-6 £29.50

Edwards, S.
Neurological physiotherapy
Churchill Liv 212pp Paperback 1996
0-443-04887-8 £19.95

Engstrom, B.
Therapy for amputees
Churchill Liv 352pp 3e. Hardback 1999
0-443-05975-6 £32.00

Hollis, M.
Massage for therapists
Blackwell Science UK 174pp 2e. Paperback 1998
0-632-04788-7 £16.99

Hollis, M.
Practical exercise therapy
Blackwell Science UK 288pp 4e. Paperback 1999
0-632-04973-1 £19.99

Hutson, M.A.
Back pain: recognition and management
Butterworth-Heinemann 224pp Hardback 1993
0-7506-0578-2 £45.00

Jones, D.
Cardiac rehabilitation
BMJ Books 264pp Hardback 1995
0-7279-0852-9 £32.00

Jones, K.
Human movement explained
Butterworth-Heinemann 384pp Paperback 1995
0-7506-1747-0 £22.50

Kesson, M.
Orthopaedic medicine: a practical approach
Butterworth-Heinemann 416pp Paperback 1998
0-7506-2543-0 £29.99

Kuprian, W.
Physical therapy for sports
W B Saunders 512pp 2e. Hardback 1995
0-7216-3758-2 £42.95

Maitland, G.D.
Peripheral manipulation
Butterworth-Heinemann 336pp Paperback 1991
0-7506-1031-X £35.00

Maitland, G.D.
Maitland's vertebral manipulation
Butterworth-Heinemann 480pp 6e. Paperback 2000
0-7506-2447-7 £37.50

Myers, R.S.
Saunders manual of physical therapy practice
W B Saunders 1426pp Hardback 1995
0-7216-3671-3 £60.00

Norris, C.M.
Sports injuries: diagnosis and management
Butterworth-Heinemann 368pp 2e. Paperback 1998
0-7506-2873-1 £34.50

Palastanga, N.
Anatomy and human movement
Butterworth-Heinemann 870pp 3e. Paperback 1998
0-7506-3268-2 £45.00

Pickles, B.
Physiotherapy with older people
Bailliere Tindall 450pp Paperback 1995
0-7020-1931-3 £38.95

Polden, M.
Physiotherapy in obstetrics and gynecology
Butterworth-Heinemann 441pp Paperback 1990
0-7506-0016-0 £32.50

Pryor, J.A.
Physiotherapy for respiratory and cardiac problems
Churchill Liv 540pp 2e. Paperback 1998
0-443-05841-5 £23.95

Reed, A.
Electrotherapy explained
Butterworth-Heinemann 400pp 3e. Paperback 2000
0-7506-4149-5 £25.00

Shepherd, R.
Physiotherapy in paediatrics
Butterworth-Heinemann 352pp 3e. Paperback 1995
0-7506-0620-7 £32.50

Swain, J.
Therapy and learning difficulties: advocacy, participation and partnership
Butterworth-Heinemann 288pp Paperback 1999
0-7506-3962-8 £25.00

Tidswell, M.
Orthopaedic physiotherapy
Mosby 264pp Paperback 1998
0-7234-2592-2 £19.95

Walker, J.M.
Physical therapy in arthritis
W B Saunders 452pp Hardback 1996
0-7216-4999-8 £44.95

Wittink, H.
Chronic pain management for physical therapy
Butterworth-Heinemann 300pp Paperback 1997
0-7506-9740-7 £35.00

PLASTIC SURGERY
(See also Surgery)

Aston, S.J.
Grabb and Smith's plastic surgery
Williams and Wilkins 1156pp 5e. Mixed-media pack 1997
0-316-32255-5 £103.50

Barrett, B.M.
Patient care in plastic surgery
Mosby 687pp 2e. Hardback 1995
0-8151-0563-0 £49.95

Georgiade, G.S.
Plastic, maxillofacial and reconstructive surgery
Williams and Wilkins 1250pp 3e. Hardback 1997
0-683-03455-3 £139.00

Marks, M.W.
Fundamentals of plastic surgery
W B Saunders 416pp Hardback 1997
0-7216-6449-0 £59.00

Masquelet, A.C.
An atlas of flaps in limb reconstruction
Martin Dunitz 280pp Hardback 1995
1-85317-172-7 £99.50

McGregor, A.
Fundamental techniques of plastic surgery
Churchill Liv 244pp 10e. Paperback 2000
0-443-063729-9 £49.95

Saffar, P.
Current practice in hand surgery
Martin Dunitz 456pp Hardback 1997
1-85317-349-5 £75.00

Settle, J.
Principles and practice of burns management
Churchill Liv 496pp Hardback 1996
0-443-04476-7 £116.00

Weinzweig, J.
Plastic surgery secrets
Hanley Belfus 750 pp Paperback 1998
1-56053-219-X £33.00

PODIATRY

Adelaar, R.S.
Hallux valgus and related disorders of the great toe
Am Ac Ortho Surgeons 100pp Paperback 1997
0-89203-168-9 £13.95

Alexander, I.J.
The foot
Churchill Liv 195pp 2e. Paperback 1997
0-443-07656-1 £25.00

Baran, R.
Diseases of the nails and their management
Blackwell Science UK 528pp 2e. Hardback 1994
0-632-03754-7 £97.50

Baxter, D.E.
The foot and ankle in sport
Mosby 400pp Hardback 1995
0-8016-6890-5 £116.00

Butterworth, R.F.
A colour atlas and text of forefoot surgery
Mosby 272pp Hardback 1990
0-7234-0991-9 £75.00

Crim, J.
Imaging of the foot and ankle
Martin Dunitz 256pp Hardback 1995
1-85317-219-7 £75.00

Donatelli, R.
The biomechanics of the foot and ankle
F A Davis 300pp 2e. Hardback 1995
0-8036-0031-3 £38.00

Helah, B.M.F.F.
Surgery of disorders of the foot and ankle
Martin Dunitz 700pp Hardback 1996
1-85317-212-X £160.00

Jahss, M.H.
Disorders of the foot: medical and surgical management
3 vols W B Saunders 3274pp Hardback 1991
0-7216-1327-6 £338.00

Jeffcoate, W.
The diabetic foot
Arnold 192pp Hardback 1995
0-412-54410-5 £85.00

Klenerman, L.
The foot and its disorders
Blackwell Science UK 512pp 3e. Hardback 1991
0-632-02951-X £89.50

Levin, M.E.
The diabetic foot
Mosby UK 656pp 5e. Hardback 1993
0-8016-6878-6 £105.00

Lorimer, D.L.
Neale's common foot disorders
Churchill Liv 496pp 5e. Hardback 1997
0-443-05258-1 £36.95

Mandel, S.
Handbook of lower extremity neurology
Churchill Liv 256pp Paperback 1999
0-443-07548-4 £39.95

Masquelet, A.C.
An atlas of surgical exposures of the lower extremity
Martin Dunitz 486pp Hardback 1993
1-85317-003-8 £149.50

McGlamry, E.D.
Comprehensive textbook of foot surgery
2 vols Williams and Wilkins 2000pp 2e.
Hardback 1992
0-683-05857-6 £300.00

McMinn, R.M.H.
Colour atlas of foot and ankle anatomy
Mosby 120pp 2e. Hardback 1995
0-7234-1995-7 £23.95

Merriman, L.M.
Assessment of the lower limb
Churchill Liv 437pp Paperback 1995
0-443-05030-9 £34.95

Mow, V.C.
Basic orthopaedic biomechanics
Williams and Wilkins 528pp 2e. Hardback 1997
0-397-51684-3 £70.00

Nicholas, J.A.
The extremities and spine in sports medicine
2 vols Mosby 1808pp 2e. Hardback 1995
0-8151-6391-6 £209.00

Philps, J.W.
The functional foot orthosis
Churchill Liv 216pp 2e. Paperback 1995
0-443-04991-2 £29.95

Redford, J.B.
Orthotics
Churchill Liv 450pp Paperback 1996
0-443-08992-2 £34.95

Rose, J.
Human walking
Williams and Wilkins 224pp 2e. Hardback 1994
0-683-07360-5 £58.00

Tibbs, D.
Varicose veins, venous disorders, and lymphatic problems in the lower limbs
Oxford UP Aus & NZ 264pp Hardback 1997
0-19-262762-7 £99.50

Tollafield, D.R.
Clinical skills in treating the foot
Churchill Liv 422pp Paperback 1997
0-443-05033-3 £34.95

Valmassy, R.L.
Clinical biomechanics of the lower extremity
Mosby 528pp Paperback 1995
0-8016-7986-9 £63.95

Whittle, M.
Gait analysis
Butterworth-Heinemann 288pp Paperback 1996
0-7506-2222-9 £19.99

Williams, G.
Chronic complications of diabetes
Blackwell Science UK 336pp Hardback 1994
0-632-03795-4 £45.00

Zatouroff, M.
A colour atlas of the foot in clinical diagnosis
Mosby 320pp Hardback 1991
0-7234-0813-0 £36.95

PSYCHIATRY
(See also Forensic Medicine & Medical Law)

Abrams, R.
Electroconvulsive therapy
Oxford UP Inc 392pp 3e. Hardback 1997
0-19-510944-9 £47.50

American Psychiatric Association
Diagnostic and statistical manual of mental disorders
Gaskell 620pp 4e. 1994
0-89042-061-0 Hardback £51.95
0-89042-062-9 Paperback £39.95

Barker, P.
Basic child psychiatry
Blackwell Science UK 379pp 6e. Paperback 1995
0-632-03772-5 £19.99

Barker, P.
Basic family therapy
Blackwell Science UK 308pp 4e. Paperback 1998
0-632-04259-1   £19.99

Barraclough, J.
Hughes' outline of modern psychiatry
John Wiley Ltd 312pp 4e. Paperback 1996
0-471-96358-5   £27.50

Bartlett, P.
Mental health law policy and practice
Blackstone Press 526pp Paperback 1999
1-85431-941-8   £24.95

Bhugra, D.
Ethnicity: an agenda for mental health
Gaskell 240pp Paperback 1999
1-901242-15-3   £25.00

Bird, J.M.
Examination notes in psychiatry
Butterworth-Heinemann 358pp 3e. Paperback 1995
0-7506-1427-7   £22.50

Bloch, S.
Introduction to the psychotherapies
Oxford UP 376pp 3e. 1996
0-19-262710-4 Hardback   £39.50
0-19-262709-0 Paperback   £19.95

British Medical Association
**Assessment of mental capacity - guidance for
doctors and lawyers**
BMA Professional Division Publications 52pp
Paperback 1995
0-7279-0913-4   £8.95

Burns, A.
Assessment scales in old age psychiatry
Martin Dunitz Hardback 1999
1-85317-562-5   £24.95

Campbell, R.J.
Psychiatric dictionary
Oxford UP Inc 824pp Hardback 1996
0-19-510259-2   £52.50

Davies, T.
ABC of mental health
BMJ Books 93pp Paperback 1998
0-7279-1220-8   £16.95

Fraser, W.I.
**Hallas' the care of people with intellectual
disabilities**
Butterworth-Heinemann 416pp 9e. Paperback 1997
0-7506-2653-4   £22.50

Freeman, C.P.
The ECT handbook
Royal Coll Psychiat 176pp Paperback 1995
0-902241-83-4   £14.99

Gelenberg, A.J.
The Practitioner's Guide to Psychoactive Drugs
Kluwer/Plenum Publ 536pp Paperback 1997
0-306-45468-8   £42.25

Gelder, M.
New Oxford textbook of psychiatry
2 vols Oxford UP 2064pp Hardback 2000
0-19-262970-0   £175.00

Gelder, M.
Psychiatry
Oxford UP 448pp 2e.1998
0-19-262887-9 Hardback   £45.00
0-19-262888-7 Paperback   £19.95

Goldberg, D.
Psychiatry in medical practice
Routledge 368pp 2e. Paperback 1994
0-415-10612-5   £17.99

Goodman, R.
Child psychiatry
Blackwell Science UK 336pp Paperback 1997
0-632-03885-3   £18.99

Goodwin, D.W.
Psychiatric diagnosis
Oxford UP 380pp 5e. 1996
0-19-510421-8 Hardback   £37.50
0-19-510422-6 Paperback   £19.95

Graham, P.
Child psychiatry
Oxford UP 576pp 3e. Paperback 1999
0-19-262864-X   £32.50

Guthrie, E.
Seminars in liaison psychiatry
Gaskell 312pp Paperback 1996
0-902241-95-8   £15.00

Harrison, P.
Lecture notes on psychiatry
Blackwell Science 198pp 8e. Paperback 1998
0-632-03677-X   £14.95

Hirsch, S.
Schizophrenia
Blackwell Science UK 760pp Hardback 1995
0-632-03276-6   £82.50

Hughes, P.
Dynamic psychotherapy explained
Radcliffe Medical 160pp Paperback 1999
1-85775-336-4   £16.95

Jacoby, R.
Psychiatry in the elderly
Oxford UP 814pp 2e. 1996
0-19-262789-9 Hardback   £99.50
0-19-262788-0 Paperback   £49.50

Johnstone, E.C.
Companion to psychiatric studies
Churchill Liv 932pp 6e. Hardback 1998
0-443-05782-6   £69.50

Kaplan, H.I.
Comprehensive textbook of psychiatry
Williams and Wilkins 7e. Hardback 1999
0-683-30128-4   £150.00

Kaplan, H.I.
Kaplan and Sadock's synopsis of psychiatry
Williams and Wilkins 1280pp 8e. Hardback 1998
0-683-30330-9   £49.95

Katona, C.
Psychiatry at a glance
Blackwell Science UK 96pp 2e. Paperback 2000
0-632-05554-5   £11.95

Kendall, P.C.
Childhood disorders
Psychology Press 240pp 2000
0-86377-608-6 Hardback   £24.95
0-86377-609-4 Paperback   £11.95

Lader, M.
Biological treatments in psychiatry
Oxford UP 458pp 2e. Hardback 1995
0-19-262652-3   £32.50

Leonard, B.
Fundamentals of psychopharmacology
John Wiley Ltd 408pp 2e. Paperback 1997
0-471-96115-9   £27.50

Leonard, B.E.
Differential effects of antidepressants
Martin Dunitz 120pp Paperback 1999
1-85317-657-5   £12.95

Levi, M.I.
Basic notes in psychiatry
Petroc Press 108pp 2e. Paperback 1998
1-900603-30-6   £12.95

Lishman, W.A.
Organic psychiatry
Blackwell Science UK 952pp 3e. Paperback 1997
0-86542-820-4   £55.00

Malhi, G.S.
Examination notes in psychiatry - basic sciences
Butterworth-Heinemann 256pp Paperback 1999
0-7506-4088-X   £17.99

Maxwell, H.
Clinical psychotherapy for health professionals
Whurr Publishers 190pp 3e. Paperback 2000
1-86156-139-3   £19.50

Murray, R.
The essentials of postgraduate psychiatry
Cambridge UP 869pp 3e. 1997
0-521-44396-2 Hardback   £105.00
0-521-57801-9 Paperback   £39.95

Puri, B.K.
Psychiatry vade-mecum
Arnold 342pp Paperback 1998
0-340-69171-9   £14.99

Puri, B.K.
Revision notes in psychiatry
Arnold 2e. Paperback 2000
0-340-76131-8   £35.00

Puri, B.K.
Textbook of psychiatry
Churchill Liv 432pp Paperback 1996
0-443-04911-4   £19.95

Rees, L.
Textbook of psychiatry
Arnold 254pp Paperback 1996
0-340-57195-0   £16.99

Reform of the Mental Health Act
Stationery Office 93pp Paperback 1999
0-10-144802-3   £10.50

Rutter, S.M.
Child and adolescent psychiatry
Blackwell Science UK 1136pp 3e. Paperback 1995
0-632-02821-1   £65.00

Sims, A.
Symptoms in the mind
W B Saunders 422pp 2e. Paperback 1995
0-7020-1788-4   £29.95

Stein, G.
Seminars in general adult psychiatry
2 vols Gaskell 1536pp Paperback 1998
0-902241-91-5   £55.00

Tyrer, P.
Drugs in psychiatric practice
ButterworthHeinemann 512pp Paperback 1997
0-7506-2251-2   £27.50

Tyrer, P.
Personality disorders
Butterworth-Heinemann 240pp 2e. Paperback 2000
0-7506-3433-2   £25.00

World Health Organization
The ICD-10 classification of mental and behavioural disorders
World Health Organization 370pp Paperback 1992
92-4-154422-8   £31.00

PSYCHOLOGY

Adams, B.
Psychology for health care
Macmillan Press Ltd 392pp 1998
0-333-64808-0 Hardback £47.50
0-333-64809-9 Paperback £15.99

Atkinson, R.
Hilgard's introduction to psychology
Harcourt College 779pp 13e. Hardback 1999
0-15-508044-X £23.95

Baum, A.
Cambridge handbook of psychology, health and medicine
Cambridge UP 678pp Paperback 1997
0-521-43686-9 £50.00

Davison, G.C.
Abnormal psychology
John Wiley Inc 720pp 8e. Hardback 2000
0-471-31811-6 £27.50

Eysenck, M.
Cognitive psychology
Psychology Press 560pp 4e. 2000
0-86377-550-0 Hardback £49.95
0-86377-551-9 Paperback £19.95

Glassman, W.E.
Approaches to psychology
Open UP 480pp 3e. Paperback 2000
0-335-20545-3 £17.99

Gross, R.
Psychology: science of mind and behaviour
Hodder Educational 959pp 3e. Paperback 1996
0-340-64762-0 £21.99

Kent, G.
Psychology and medical care
W B Saunders Co Ltd 240pp 3e. Paperback 1996
0-7020-2065-6 £16.95

Malim, T.
Introductory psychology
Macmillan Press Ltd 1024pp Paperback 1998
0-333-66852-9 £19.99

Mayhew, J.
Psychological change
Macmillan Press Ltd 264pp 1997
0-333-65430-7 Hardback £45.00
0-333-65431-5 Paperback £14.99

Messer, D.
Psychology for nurses and health care professionals
Harvester Wheatsheaf 480pp Paperback 1995
0-13-433178-8 £18.99

Oatley, K.
Understanding emotions
Blackwell Publishers 459pp Paperback 1995
1-55786-495-0 £16.99

Ogden, J.
Health psychology
Open UP 384pp 2e. 2000
0-335-20597-6 Hardback £55.00
0-335-20596-8 Paperback £17.99

Parkin, A.J.
Essentials of cognitive psychology
Psychology Press 352pp 2000
0-86377-672-8 Hardback £34.95
0-86377-673-6 Paperback £13.95

Porter, M.
Psychology and sociology applied to medicine
Churchill Liv 174pp Paperback 1998
0-443-04971-8 £17.95

Sarafino, E.P.
Health psychology
Wiley 599pp Hardback 1998
0-471-16917-X £24.95

Stroebe, W.
Social psychology and health
Open UP 288pp 2e. Paperback 2000
0-335-19922-4 Hardback £50.00
0-335-19921-6 Paperback £16.99

Walsh, K.W.
Neuropsychology
Churchill Liv 492pp 4e. Paperback 1999
0-443-06051-7 £29.50

Wilkinson, J.D.
Psychology in counselling and therapeutic practice
John Wiley Ltd 286pp Paperback 1997
0-471-95562-0 £19.99

PUBLIC HEALTH & SOCIAL MEDICINE
(See also Epidemiology)

Abramson, J.H.
Survey methods in community medicine
Churchill Liv 440pp 5e. Paperback 1999
0-443-06163-7 £22.95

Acheson, D.
Independent inquiry into inequalities in health
Stationery Office Paperback 1998
0-11-322173-8 £19.50

Armstrong, D.
An outline of sociology as applied to medicine
Butterworth-Heinemann 164pp 4e. Hardback 1995
0-7506-1929-5 £15.50

Bassett, W.H.
Clay's handbook of environmental health
E & FN Spon 968pp 18e. Hardback 1999
0-419-22960-4   £99.00

Baxter, P.
Hunter's diseases of occupation
Arnold 1000pp 9e. Hardback 1999
0-340-67750-3   £155.00

Beaglehole, R.
Public health at the crossroads
Cambridge UP 261pp Paperback 1997
0-521-58665-8   £21.95

Bowling, A.
Measuring disease
Open UP 400pp Paperback 1995
0-335-19225-4   £22.50

Bowling, A.
Measuring health
Open UP 256pp 2e. Paperback 1997
0-335-19754-X   £17.99

Connelly, J.
Making sense of public health medicine
Radcliffe Medical 160pp Paperback 1997
1-85775-186-8   £18.95

Davies, B.M.
Public health, preventive medicine and social services
Arnold 432pp 6e. Paperback 1995
0-340-61373-4   £14.99

Department of Health
On the state of the public health
Stationery Office Paperback 1998
0-11-322113-4   £18.50

Department of Health
Our healthier nation
Stationery Office 174pp Paperback 1999
0-10-143862-1   £15.00

Department of Health
Smoking kills
Stationery Office 100pp Paperback 1998
0-10-141772-1   £11.50

Detels, R.
Oxford textbook of public health
3 vols Oxford UP 1646pp 3e. Hardback 1996
0-19-262553-5   £195.00

Donaldson, L.J.
Essential public health medicine
Petroc Press 384pp 2e. Paperback 1999
1-900603-32-2   £24.95

Farmer, R.
Lecture notes on epidemiology and public health medicine
Blackwell Science UK 296pp 4e. Paperback 1996
0-86542-611-2   £15.95

Griffiths, S.
Perspectives in public health
Radcliffe Medical 296pp Paperback 1999
1-85775-209-0   £25.00

Kloss, D.
Occupational health law
Blackwell Science UK 400pp 3e. Hardback 1998
0-632-04263-X   £49.50

Marmot, M.
Social determinants of health
Oxford UP 306pp Paperback 1999
0-19-263069-5   £26.50

McDonald, C.
Epidemiology of work related diseases
BMJ Books 567pp 2e. Paperback 1999
0-7279-1432-4   £65.00

Parkes, W.R.
Occupational lung disorders
Butterworth-Heinemann 576pp 3e. Hardback 1994
0-7506-1403-X   £190.00

Scambler, G.B.P.
Sociology as applied to medicine
W B Saunders 352pp 4e. Paperback 1997
0-7020-2275-6   £14.95

Seaton, A.
Practical occupational medicine
Arnold 288pp Paperback 1994
0-340-55936-5   £35.00

Snashall, D.
ABC of work related disorders
BMJ Books 79pp Paperback 1997
0-7279-1154-6   £15.95

Waldron, H.A.
Occupational health practice
Butterworth-Heinemann 352pp 4e. Hardback 1997
0-7506-2720-4   £57.50

RADIOLOGY & RADIOGRAPHY

Allan, P.
Clinical Doppler ultrasound
Churchill Liv 256pp Paperback 2000
0-443-05549-1   £44.95

Ansell, G.
Complications in diagnostic imaging and interventional radiology
Blackwell Science USA 736pp 3e.Hardback 1996
0-86542-243-5 £160.00

Armstrong, P.
Diagnostic and interventional radiology in surgical practice
Arnold 608pp 1997
0-412-61960-1 Hardback £100.00
0-412-61970-9 Paperback £60.00

Armstrong, P.
Diagnostic imaging
Blackwell Science USA 472pp 4e. Hardback 1998
0-86542-696-1 £29.95

Armstrong, P.
Imaging of diseases of the chest
Mosby 1056pp 3e. Hardback 2000
0-7234-3166-3 £150.00

Ball, J.
Essential physics for radiographers
Blackwell Science UK 400pp 3e. Paperback 1997
0-632-03902-7 £19.99

Ball, J.L.
Chesney's radiographic imaging
Blackwell Science UK 448pp 6e.Hardback 1995
0-632-03901-9 £24.95

Bushong, S.C.
Radiation protection
McGraw-Hill USA 288pp Paperback 1998
0-07-012013-7 £22.99

Callen, P.W.
Ultrasonography in Obs/Gyn
W B Saunders 4e. Hardback 2000
0-7216-8132-8 £65.00

Carter, P.R.
Chesney's equipment for student radiographers
Blackwell Science UK 336pp 4e. Paperback 1994
0-632-02724-X £22.99

Chapman, S.
Aids to radiological differential diagnosis
W B Saunders Co Ltd 576pp 3e. Paperback 1995
0-7020-1895-3 £19.95

Chapman, S.
A guide to radiological procedures
W B Saunders Co Ltd 448pp 4e. Paperback 2000
0-7020-2565-8 £19.95

Corne, J.
Chest x-ray made easy
Churchill Liv 128pp Paperback 1997
0-443-05194-1 £11.95

Culmer, P.
Chesney's care of the patient in diagnostic radiography
Blackwell Science UK 304pp 7e. Paperback 1995
0-632-03762-8 £16.99

Curati, W.
Imaging in oncology
Greenwich Medical 230pp Paperback 1998
1-900151-03-0 £24.50

Delchar, T.A.
Physics in medical diagnosis
Kluwer Academic Publ 376pp Paperback 1996
0-412-61680-7 £60.50

Dendy, P.P.
Physics for diagnostic radiology
IOP 416pp 2e. Paperback 1999
0-7503-0591-6 £29.00

Farr, R.F.
Physics for medical imaging
Bailliere Tindall 288pp Paperback 1996
0-7020-1770-1 £25.95

Graham, D.T.
Principles of radiological physics
Churchill Liv 667pp Paperback 1996
0-443-04816-9 £38.95

Grainger, R.G.
Diagnostic radiology
3 vols Churchill Liv 3000pp 3e. Hardback 1996
0-443-05167-4 £310.00

Hare, W.
Clinical radiology for medical students and health practitioners
Blackwell Science 285pp Paperback 1999
0-86793-007-1 £22.95

Henwood, S.
Clinical CT - techniques and practice
Greenwich Medical 132pp Paperback 1999
1-900151-56-1 £17.50

Keats, T.E.
Atlas of normal roentgen variants that may simulate disease
Mosby 1042pp 6e. Hardback 1996
0-8151-4951-4 £179.00

Kirkwood, J.R.
Essentials of neuroimaging
Churchill Liv 752pp 2e. Hardback 1995
0-443-08946-9 £111.00

Lee, L.
Fundamentals of mammography
W B Saunders Co Ltd 160pp Paperback 1995
0-7020-1797-3 £32.95

Lisle, D.
Imaging for students
Arnold 192pp Paperback 1995
0-340-61383-1   £18.99

Maisey, M.N.
Clinical nuclear medicine
Arnold 768pp 3e. Hardback 1998
0-412-75180-1   £150.00

Martin, J.
Physics of radiation protection
John Wiley Inc 832pp Hardback 2000
0-471-35373-6   £96.95

Martin, A.
An introduction to radiation protection
Arnold 240pp 4e. Paperback 1996
0-412-63110-5   £22.50

Nias, A.H.W.
An introduction to radiobiology
John Wiley Ltd 400pp 2e. Paperback 1998
0-471-97590-7   £32.50

Novelline, R.A.
Squire's fundamentals of radiology
Harvard UP 632pp 5e. Hardback 1997
0-674-83339-2   £45.50

Patel, P.R.
Lecture notes on radiology
Blackwell Science UK 288pp Paperback 1997
0-632-04758-5   £14.95

Paterson, A.
Clinical radiography
Isis Medical Media 350pp Hardback 2000
1-899066-51-9   £45.00

Perkins, A.C.
Nuclear medicine therapy
John Libbey 200pp Hardback 2000
0-86196-570-1   £28.00

Ray, K.K.
An aid to radiology for the MRCP
Blackwell Science UK 288pp Paperback 2000
0-632-04912-X   £22.50

Roberts, G.M.
Clinical radiology for medical students
Butteworth-Heinemann 160pp 3e. Paperback 1998
0-7506-1408-0   £17.50

Scally, P.
Medical imaging
Oxford UP 302pp Paperback 1999
0-19-263056-3   £19.95

Sharp, P.F.
Practical nuclear medicine
Oxford UP 362pp 2e. 1998
0-19-262842-9 Hardback   £65.00
0-19-262841-0 Paperback   £32.50

Steel, G.G.
Basic clinical radiobiology
Arnold 264pp 2e. Hardback 1997
0-340-70020-3   £34.99

Sutton, D.
Radiology and imaging for medical students
Churchill Liv 280pp 7e. Paperback 1998
0-443-05917-9   £21.95

Sutton, D.
Textbook of radiology and imaging
Churchill Liv 1600pp 6e.Hardback 1997
0-443-05368-5   £279.00

Webb, W.R.
Fundamentals of body CT
W B Saunders 352pp 2e. Paperback 1997
0-7216-6862-3   £34.95

Weir, J.
Atlas and text of clinical imaging
Mosby 256pp Paperback 1998
0-7234-2555-8   £23.95

Westbrook, C.
Handbook of MRI technique
Blackwell Science UK 432pp 2e. Paperback 1999
0-632-05264-3   £24.99

Westbrook, C.
MRI in practice
2e. Blackwell Science UK 336pp Paperback 1998
0-632-04205-2   £24.99

Whitehouse, G.H.
Techniques in diagnostic imaging
Blackwell Science USA 544pp 3e. Hardback 1995
0-86542-808-5   £75.00

Williamson, M.R.
Essentials of ultrasound
W B Saunders 274pp Hardback 1996
0-7216-6642-6   £36.95

REHABILITATION
(See also, Occupational Therapy, Physiotherapy)

Barnes, M.
Textbook of rehabilitation medicine
Oxford UP 404pp Paperback 2000
0-19-262805-4   £29.50

Carr, J.H.
Neurological rehabilitation
Butterworth-Heinemann 368pp Paperback 1998
0-7506-0971-0   £27.50

Chamberlain, M.A.
Traumatic brain injury rehabilitation
Stanley Thornes 288pp Paperback 1995
0-412-48970-8 £22.50

Clarke, A.
Rehabilitation techniques in rheumatology
Martin Dunitz 320pp 2e. Paperback 2001
1-85317-120-4 £29.95

Davies, P.M.
Starting again: early rehabilitation after traumatic brain injury or other severe brain lesions
Springer-Verlag Berl 370pp Paperback 1994
3-540-55934-5 £23.95

DeLisa, J.A.
Rehabilitation medicine
Williams and Wilkins 1856pp 3e. Hardback 1998
0-7817-1015-4 £115.00

Ekdawi, M.
Psychiatric rehabilitation
Stanley Thornes 160pp Paperback 1993
0-412-42970-5 £21.00

Fawcus, R.
Stroke rehabilitation
Blackwell Science UK 256pp Paperback 1999
0-632-04998-7 £22.50

Goodwill, C.J.
Rehabilitation of the physically disabled adult
Stanley Thornes 822pp 2e. Hardback 1997
0-7487-3183-0 £44.00

Hammell, K.W.
Spinal cord injury rehabilitation
Stanley Thornes 368pp Paperback 1994
0-412-47680-0 £21.00

Helewa, A.
Critical evaluation of research in physical rehabilitation: towards evidence-based practice
W B Saunders Paperback 271pp 2000
0-7216-7390-2 £23.95

Nocon, A.
Trends in rehabilitation policy
King's Fund Paperback 1998
1-85717-182-9 £5.99

Peat, M.
Community based rehabilitation
W B Saunders 300pp Hardback 1997
0-7020-1941-0 £26.95

Pitt-Brooke, J.
Rehabilitation of movement
W B Saunders 608pp Hardback 1997
0-7020-2157-1 £26.95

Ponsford, J.
Traumatic brain injury
Psychology Press 352pp Hardback 1995
0-86377-376-1 £35.00

Squires, A.J.
Rehabilitation of older people
Stanley Thornes 313pp 2e. Paperback 1996
0-412-71930-4 £21.00

Wilson, B.A.
Rehabilitation studies handbook
Cambridge UP 425pp Paperback 1997
0-521-43713-X £35.00

RESPIRATORY MEDICINE

Albert, R.K.
Comprehensive respiratory medicine
Mosby 800pp Hardback 1999
0-7234-3118-3 £99.95

Barnes, P.J.
Asthma: basic mechanisms
Academic Press 864pp 3e. Hardback 1998
0-12-079027-0 £94.95

Baum, G.L.
Textbook of pulmonary diseases
2 vols Williams and Wilkins 2040pp 6e. Paperback 1997
0-316-08434-4 £162.00

Bourke, S.J.
Lecture notes on respiratory medicine
Blackwell Science UK 216pp 5e. Paperback 1998
0-632-04968-5 £14.95

Cherniak, N.S.
Rehabilitation of the patient with respiratory disease
McGraw-Hill HPD 724pp Hardback 1999
0-07-011649-0 £119.99

Clark, T.
Asthma
Arnold 550pp Hardback 2000
0-340-76123-7 £95.00

Clark, T.
Practical management of asthma
Martin Dunitz 176pp 3e. Paperback 1998
1-85317-587-0 £29.95

Corrin, B.
Pathology of the lungs
Churchill Liv 656pp Hardback 1999
0-443-05713-3 £175.00

Cotes, J.E.
Lung function - assessment and application in medicine
Blackwell Science UK 784pp 5e. Hardback 1993
0-632-03526-9 £75.00

Davies, P.D.O.
Clinical tuberculosis
Arnold 756pp 2e. Hardback 1998
0-412-80340-2 £99.00

Harris, A.
Cystic fibrosis: the facts
Oxford Paperbacks 138pp Paperback 1995
0-19-262543-8 £9.99

Hodson, M.E.
Cystic fibrosis
Arnold 608pp 2e. Hardback 2000
0-340-74208-9 £95.00

Hughes, J.M.
Lung function tests: physiological principles and chemical applications
W B Saunders 328pp Paperback 1999
0-7020-2350-7 £25.00

James, D.G.
A colour atlas of respiratory diseases
Mosby 368pp 2e. Hardback 1992
0-7234-1695-8 £79.00

Kinnear, W.
Key topics in respiratory medicine
Bios Scientific 250pp Paperback 1998
1-85996-271-8 £18.95

Rees, J.
ABC of asthma
4e. BMJ Books 50pp Paperback 1999
0-7279-1261-5 £14.95

Russell, J.A.
Acute respiratory distress syndrome
Cambridge UP 368pp Paperback 1999
0-521-65410-6 £29.95

Seaton, A.
Crofton and Douglas's respiratory diseases
Blackwell Science UK 1666pp 5e. Hardback 2000
0-86542-857-3 £195.00

Simonds, A.K.
Pulmonary rehabilitation
BMJ Books 248pp Paperback 1996
0-7279-1022-1 £27.00

Sykes, K.
Respiratory support in intensive care
BMJ Books 315pp 2e. Paperback 1999
0-7279-1379-4 £30.00

West, J.B.
Pulmonary pathophysiology
Williams and Wilkins 193pp 5e. Paperback 1998
0-683-30225-6 £22.95

West, J.B.
Respiratory physiology: the essentials
Williams and Wilkins 250pp 6e. Paperback 1999
0-683-30734-7 £17.95

Wilkins, R.
Lung sounds
Mosby 144pp Mixed-media pack 1996
0-8151-9287-8 Paperback and cassette £37.69
0-8151-9417-X Paperback and CD £39.98

RHEUMATOLOGY
(See also Orthopaedics)

Doherty, M.
Color atlas and text of osteoarthritis
Mosby 208pp Hardback 1994
0-7234-1646-X £79.00

Doherty, M.
Rheumatology examination and injection techniques
W B Saunders 160pp 2e. Hardback 1998
0-7020-2387-6 £37.00

Ferrari, R.
Rheumatology guidebook
Bios Scientific 200pp Paperback 1996
1-85996-215-7 £19.95

Firestein, G.
Rheumatoid arthritis: new frontiers
Oxford UP 608pp Hardback 2000
0-19-262972-7 £125.00

Hughes, G.R.V.
Connective tissue diseases
Blackwell Science UK 328pp 4e. Hardback 1994
0-632-03752-0 £40.00

Ruddy, S.
Kelley's textbook of rheumatology
2 vols W B Saunders 2016pp 6e. Hardback 2000
0-7216-8008-9 £160.00

Klippel, J.H.
Practical rheumatology
Mosby 432pp Hardback 1995
0-7234-2429-2 £45.00

Klippel, J.H.:
Rheumatology
Mosby 1880pp 2e. 1997
0-7234-2405-5 Hardback £245.00
0-7234-3000-4 CD-ROM £222.08

Maddison, P.J.
Oxford textbook of rheumatology
2 vols Oxford UP 2208pp 2e. Hardback 1998
0-19-262697-3   £225.00

Moll, J.M.H.
Rheumatology
Churchill Liv 164pp 2e. Paperback 1997
0-443-05805-9   £11.95

Shipley, M.
A colour atlas of rheumatology
Mosby 176pp 3e. Hardback 1992
0-7234-1689-3   £30.00

Snaith, M.L.
ABC of rheumatology
BMJ Books 100pp 2e. Paperback 1999
0-7279-1385-9   £17.95

SEXUALLY TRANSMITTED DISEASES
(See also, AIDS & HIV, Infectious Diseases)

Adler, M.W.
ABC of sexually transmitted diseases
BMJ Books 81pp 4e. Paperback 1998
0-7279-1368-9   £16.95

Barton, S.
Handbook of genitourinary medicine
Arnold 496pp Paperback 1998
0-340-74084-1   £45.00

Handsfield, H.H.
Color atlas and synopsis of sexually transmitted diseases
McGraw-Hill HPD 250pp 2e. Paperback 1999
0-07-026033-8   £38.99

Holmes, K.K.
Sexually transmitted diseases
McGraw-Hill HPD 1440pp 3e. Hardback 1998
0-07-029688-X   £120.00

McMillan, A.
Colour guide: sexually transmitted infections
Churchill Liv 128pp 2e. Paperback 2000
0-443-06229-3   £11.95

Morse, S.A.
Atlas of sexually transmitted disease and AIDS
Mosby 400pp 2e. Hardback 1995
0-7234-2143-9   £122.00

Sonnex, C.
A general practitioner's guide to genitourinary medicine and sexual health
Cambridge UP 121pp Paperback 1996
0-521-55656-2   £18.95

Tomlinson, J.
ABC of sexual health
BMJ Books 67pp Paperback 1999
0-7279-1373-5   £14.95

Wisdom, A.
Diagnosis in colour: sexually transmitted diseases
Mosby 328pp 2e. Paperback 1997
0-7234-2496-9   £21.95

SPEECH & LANGUAGE THERAPY

Adams. C.
Assessments in speech therapy
Routledge 288pp 2e. Hardback 1993
0-415-07881-4   £47.50

Albery, L.
Cleft palate sourcebook
Winslow Press 110pp Spiralbound 1994
0-86388-127-0   £32.50

Beech, J.
Assesments in speech therapy
Routledge 288pp Paperback 1993
0-415-07882-2   £17.99

Bench, J.
Communication skills in hearing-impaired children
Whurr Publishers 343pp Paperback 1992
1-870332-38-5   £29.50

Brown, B.B.
Developmental disorders of language
Whurr Publishers 250pp Paperback 1997
1-86156-020-6   £24.50

Code, C.
Treatment of aphasia
Whurr Publishers 361pp Paperback 1995
1-870332-33-4   £24.50

Dalton, P.
Counselling people with communication problems
Sage London 176pp Paperback 1994
0-8039-8895-8   £12.99

Doyle, J.
Practical audiology for speech-language therapists
Whurr Publishers 300pp Paperback 1998
1-86156-059-1   £19.50

Duffy, J.R.
Motor speech disorders
Mosby 350pp Hardback 1995
0-8016-6944-8   £42.95

Enderby, P.
Therapy outcome measures: speech and language therapy
Singular Mixed-media pack 1997
1-56593-807-0 £34.00

Fawcus, M.
Stuttering: from theory to practice
Whurr Publishers 164pp Paperback 1995
1-897635-81-8 £22.50

Greene, M.C.L.
The voice and its disorders
Whurr Publishers 428pp 5e. 1989
1-870332-25-3 Hardback £47.50
1-870332-30-X Paperback £29.50

Grunwell, P.
Developmental speech disorders
Whurr Publishers 198pp Paperback 1990
1-897635-70-2 £29.50

Jordan, L.
Aphasia: a social approach
Stanley Thornes 232pp Paperback 1996
0-412-49700-X £16.50

Law, J.
Communication difficulties in childhood
Radcliffe Medical 360pp Paperback 1999
1-85775-098-5 £19.95

Logemann, J.A.
Evaluation and treatment of swallowing disorders
Singular 2e. Hardback 1997
0-89079-274-7 £32.95

Love, R.J.
Neurology for the Speech-Language Pathologist
Butterworth-Heinemann 384pp 4e. Paperback 2000
0-7506-7252-8 £27.50

Martin, M.
Speech audiometry
Whurr Publishers 250pp 2e. Paperback 1997
1-897635-12-5 £27.50

Martini, A.
Genetics and hearing impairment
Whurr Publishers 300pp Paperback 1996
1-897635-29-X £35.00

McCormick, B.
Paediatric audiology: 0-5 years
Whurr Publishers 458pp 2e. Paperback 1993
1-897635-25-7 £24.50

Rustin, L.
Social skills and the speech impaired
Whurr Publishers 250pp 2e. Paperback 1998
1-897635-56-7 £22.50

Snowling, M.
Dyslexia, speech and language: a practitioner's handbook
Whurr Publishers 250pp Paperback 1996
1-897635-48-6 £19.50

Van der Gaag, A.
Clinical guidelines by consensus for speech and language therapists
Royal College of Speech and Language Therapists 76pp Paperback 1998
1-947589-08-2 £10.00

Van der Gaag, A.
Communication quality 2 - professional standards for speech and language therapists
Royal College of Speech and Language Therapists 330pp 2e. Paperback 1996
0-947589-04-X £14.95

Wing, L.
The autistic spectrum: a guide for parents
Constable 208pp Hardback 1996
0-09-475160-9 £16.99

SPORTS MEDICINE

Bird, S.
Sports injuries
Stanley Thornes 264pp Paperback 1997
0-7487-3181-4 £26.50

Hackney, R.G.
Sports medicine handbook
BMJ Books 505pp Hardback 1999
0-7279-1031-0 £75.00

Harries, M.
Oxford textbook of sports medicine
Oxford UP 982pp 2e. Paperback 2000
0-19-263236-1 £49.50

Hutson, M.A.
Sports injuries: recognition and management
Oxford UP 246pp 2e. Paperback 1996
0-19-262675-2 £34.50

Kent, M.
Oxford dictionary of sports science and medicine
Oxford UP 582pp 2e. Hardback 1998
0-19-262845-3 £19.95

MacAuley, D.
The benefits and hazards of exercise
BMJ Books 394pp Paperback 1999
0-7279-1412-X £35.00

MacAuley, D.
Sports medicine: a practical guide for general practice
Butterworth-Heinemann 192pp Paperback 1998
0-7506-3730-7 £22.50

McArdle, W.D.
Exercise physiology
Williams and Wilkins 870pp 4e. Hardback 1996
0-683-05731-6   £29.95

McLatchie, G.R.
ABC of sports medicine
BMJ Books 120pp 2e. Paperback 1999
0-7279-1366-2   £18.95

McLatchie, G.R.
The soft tissue: trauma and sports injuries
Butterworth-Heinemann 496pp Paperback 1996
0-7506-3065-5   £35.00

Payne, S.D.W.
Medicine, sport & the law
Blackwell Science UK 400pp Paperback 1990
0-632-02439-9   £32.50

Read, M.
A practical guide to sports injuries
Butterworth-Heinemann 336pp Paperback 2000
0-7506-3251-8   £25.00

Read, M.
Sports injuries: a unique guide to self-diagnosis
Butterworth-Heinemann 336pp 2e. Paperback 2000
0-7506-3112-0   £13.99

Sherry, E.
Oxford handbook of sports medicine
Oxford UP 946pp Plastic-reinforced paper 1998
0-19-262890-9   £19.95

Sherry, E.
Sports medicine
Churchill Liv 122pp Paperback 1997
0-443-05482-7   £11.95

SUBSTANCE ABUSE

Beaumont, B.
Care of drug users in general practice
Radcliffe Medical 200pp Paperback 1997
1-85775-236-8   £17.95

British Medical Association
The misuse of drugs
Harwood Academic 160pp Paperback 1997
90-5702-260-5   £12.99

Cooper, D.B.
Alcohol use
Radcliffe Medical 240pp Paperback 2000
1-85775-121-3   £19.95

Department of Health
Drug misuse and dependence
Stationery Office 132pp Paperback 1999
0-11-322277-7   £9.50

Edwards, G.
The treatment of drinking problems
Cambridge UP 3e. 380pp 1997
0-521-49696-9 Hardback   £65.00
0-521-49793-0 Paperback   £24.95

Ghodse, A.H.
Drugs and addictive behaviour
Blackwell Science UK 386pp 2e. Paperback 1995
0-86542-868-9   £29.50

Gossop, M.
Living with drugs
Ashgate 192pp 5e. Paperback 2000
1-84014-939-6   £14.95

Heather, N.
Problem drinking
Oxford UP 238pp 3e.Paperback 1997
0-19-262861-5   £19.95

Keene, J.
Drug misuse
Stanley Thornes 376pp Paperback 1996
0-412-64280-8   £21.50

Robertson, J.R.
Management of drug users in the community
Arnold 432pp Paperback 1998
0-340-70013-0   £19.99

Robson, P.
Forbidden drugs
Oxford UP 208pp 2e. Paperback 1999
0-19-262955-7   £12.99

Royal College of Psychiatrists and the Royal
College of Physicians
Dilemmas and choices
Gaskell Paperback 2000
1-901242-44-7   £9.50

Society for the Study of Addiction
Tackling alcohol together
Free Assoc Books 368pp Paperback 1999
1-85343-458-2   £15.95

Tackling drugs to build a better Britain
Stationery Office 36pp Paperback 1998
0-10-139452-7   £6.50

Walle, T.A.N.
Treating problem drinkers and drug misuers in the community
Blackwell Publishers 288pp 2e. Paperback 1999
0-632-03575-7   £19.99

Wills, S.
Drugs of abuse
Pharmaceutical Press 273pp Paperback 1997
0-85369-352-8   £16.95

SURGERY
(See also Plastic Surgery)

al-Fallouji, M.
Postgraduate surgery: the candidate's guide
Butterworth-Heinemann 624pp 2e. Paperback 1998
0-7506-1591-5   £75.00

Beard, J.D.
Vascular and endovascular surgery
W B Saunders 420pp Hardback 1998
0-7020-2145-8   £48.00

Brown, T.H.
Introduction to minimal access surgery
BMJ Books 100pp Paperback 1996
0-7279-0885-5   £30.00

Browse, N.
An introduction to the symptoms and signs of surgical disease
Arnold 464pp 3e. Paperback 1997
0-340-66211-5   £24.99

Burkitt, H.G.
Essential surgery
2e. Churchill Liv 756pp Paperback 1995
0-443-04805-3   £36.95

Burnand, K.G.
The new Aird's companion in surgical studies
Churchill Liv 1248pp 2e. Hardback 1998
0-443-05326-X   £95.00

Carter, D.C.
Atlas of general surgery
Arnold 1208pp 3e.Hardback 1996
0-412-72090-6   £95.00

Carter, D.C.
Hepatobiliary and pancreatic surgery
Arnold 688pp Hardback 1996
0-412-61930-X   £210.00

Cuschieri, A.
Essential surgical practice
Butterworth-Heinemann 600pp Hardback 2000
0-7506-4780-9   £65.00

Cuschieri, A.
Clinical surgery
Vol.1 Blackwell Science UK 608pp 4e.
Paperback 1996
0-632-03146-8   £29.50

Dent, J.
Surgery 2
Churchill Liv 232pp Paperback 1997
0-443-05171-2   £16.95

Dunn, D.C.
Surgical diagnosis and management
Blackwell Science USA 640pp Paperback 1999
0-86542-718-6   £22.50

Ellis, B.W.
Hamilton Bailey's emergency surgery
Arnold 880pp 13e. Hardback 2000
0-340-76380-9   £95.00

Ellis, H.
French's index of surgical differential diagnosis
Butterworth-Heinemann 464pp 1999
0-7506-2763-8   £35.00

Ellis, H.
Lecture notes on general surgery
Blackwell Science UK 416pp 9e. Paperback 1998
0-86542-768-2   £15.95

Farndon, J.R.
Breast and endocrine surgery
W B Saunders Co Ltd 350pp Hardback 1997
0-7020-2144-X   £49.95

Fligelstone, L.
Essential postgraduate surgery
Churchill Liv 352pp Paperback 2000
0-443-06025-8   £25.00

Forrest, A.P.M.
Principles and practice of surgery
Churchill Liv 642pp 3e. Paperback 1995
0-443-04860-6   £39.00

Forsythe, J.L.R.
Transplantation surgery
W B Saunders 352pp Hardback 1997
0-7020-2146-6   £48.00

Gardner, D.
Pathology for surgeons in training
Arnold 416pp 2e. Paperback 1996
0-340-60374-7   £30.00

Gompertz, R.H.K.
Churchill's house surgeon's survival guide
Churchill Liv 352pp 2e. Paperback 2000
0-443-06223-4   £16.95

Greig, J.D.
Color atlas of general surgical diagnosis
Mosby 346pp 2e. Hardback 1996
0-7234-2057-2   £29.95

Hambly, P.R.
Perioperative management for house surgeons
Bios Scientific 240pp Paperback 1996
1-85996-185-1   £17.95

Hargreaves, D.H.
On-the-job training for surgeons
Royal Soc Medicine 132pp Paperback 1997
1-85315-314-1   £17.50

Hobsley, M.
Pathways in surgery
Arnold 500pp 3e. Paperback 2001
0-340-63186-4   £24.99

Jamieson, C.W.
Rob and Smith's operative surgery: concise vascular surgery
Arnold 352pp Hardback 1997
0-412-82450-7   £65.00

Johnson, C.
Essential surgical technique
Arnold 328pp Paperback 1997
0-412-55470-4   £27.00

Keen, G.
Operative surgery and management
Butterworth-Heinemann 976pp 3e. Paperback 1998
0-7506-4238-6   £65.00

Kirk, R.M.
Basic surgical techniques
Churchill Liv 192pp 4e. Paperback 1995
0-443-05065-1   £29.95

Kirk, R.M.
Clinical surgery in general
Churchill Liv 464pp 3e. Paperback 1999
0-443-06219-6   £47.95

Kirk, R.M.
General surgical operations
Churchill Liv 879pp 3e. Hardback 1994
0-443-04715-4   £105.00

Lavelle-Jones, M.
Surgery - 1
Churchill Liv 207pp Paperback 1996
0-443-05172-0   £16.95

Lumley, J.S.P.
Hamilton Bailey's demonstration of physical signs in clinical surgery
Butterworth-Heinemann 512pp 18e. Paperback 1997
0-7506-1621-0   £39.50

McLatchie, G.R.
Oxford handbook of operative surgery
Oxford UP 734pp Paperback 1996
0-19-262097-5   £18.95

Morris, P.J.
Oxford textbook of surgery
Oxford UP 2500pp 2e. Hardback 2000
0-19-262884-4   £325.00

Mowschenson, P.M.
Aids to undergraduate surgery
Churchill Liv 163pp 4e. Paperback 1994
0-443-04966-1   £12.95

Paterson-Brown, S.
Emergency surgery and critical care
W B Saunders 326pp Hardback 1997
0-7020-2140-7   £49.00

Pollock, D.J.
Surgical pathology
Arnold 496pp Hardback 2000
0-340-74099-X   £65.00

Poston, G.J.
Principles of operative surgery
Churchill Liv 246pp 2e. Paperback 1996
0-443-05019-8   £19.95

Quick, C.
Principles of surgical management
Oxford UP 528pp Hardback 2000
0-19-262230-7   £79.50

Rintoul, R.F.
Farquharson's textbook of operative surgery
Churchill Liv 714pp 8e. Hardback 1995
0-443-04712-X   £90.00

Russell, R.C.G.
Bailey and Love's short practice of surgery
Arnold 1184pp 23e. Hardback 2000
0-340-75924-0   £85.00

Sabiston Jr, D.C.
Textbook of modern surgery
W B Saunders 2352pp 15e. Hardback 1996
0-7216-5887-3   £85.00

Schwartz, S.I.
Principles of surgery
McGraw-Hill USA 2176pp 7e. Hardback 1998
0-07-054256-2   £81.99

Smith, J.M.B.
The surgeon's guide to antimicrobial chemotherapy
Arnold 286pp Hardback 2000
0-340-74196-1   £29.99

Spitz, L.
Rob and Smith's operative surgery: concise pediatric surgery
Arnold 360pp Hardback 1997
0-412-82780-8   £70.00

Taylor, I.
Surgical principles
Arnold 224pp Paperback 1996
0-340-61379-3   £35.00

Williamson, R.C.N.
Scott: an aid to clinical surgery
Churchill Liv 400pp 6e. Paperback 1998
0-443-05603-X   £17.95

TROPICAL MEDICINE

Bell, D.
Lecture notes on tropical medicine
Blackwell Science UK 384pp 4e. Paperback 1995
0-632-03839-X   £15.95

Burns, A.A.
Where women have no doctor: health guide for women
Macmillan Education 596pp 1997
0-333-64933-8   £7.99

CAB International/Wellcome Trust
Topics in international health series on CD-ROM
CAB International 1998
See website for information: http://www.cabi.org

Canizares, O.
A manual of dermatology for developing countries
Oxford UP 380pp Hardback 1993
0-19-262293-5   £57.00

Cheesbrough, M.
District laboratory practice in tropical countries
Cambridge UP 462pp Paperback 1999
0-521-66547-7   £35.00

Chiodini, P.
Blacklock and Southwell's human parasitology
Kluwer Academic Publ 400pp 11e. Hardback 1996
0-412-43480-6   £65.00

Cook, G.
Manson's tropical diseases
W B Saunders Co Ltd 1824pp 20e. Hardback 1995
0-7020-1764-7   £100.00

Cox, F.
Topley and Wilson's microbiology and microbial infection. Vol. 5: Parasitology
Arnold 701pp 9e. Hardback 1998
0-340-66320-0   £125.00

Crofton, J.
Clinical tuberculosis
Macmillan Heinemann 240pp Paperback 1998
0-333-72430-5   £5.00

Doerr, W.
Tropical pathology
Springer-Verlag Berl 1105pp 2e. Hardback 1995
3-540-59391-8   £346.00

Ebrahim, G.J.
Paediatric practice in developing countries
Macmillan Education 352pp 2e. Paperback 1993
0-333-57347-1   £16.75

Eddleston, M.
Oxford handbook of tropical medicine
Oxford UP 666pp Paperback 1999
0-19-262772-4   £19.95

Gilles, H.M.
Bruce-Chwatt's essential malariology
Arnold 360pp 3e. Paperback 1993
0-340-57190-X   £59.50

Gilles, H.M.
Protozoal diseases
Arnold 768pp Hardback 1999
0-340-74090-6   £145.00

Gillespie, S.
Medical parasitology: a practical approach
Oxford UP 314pp 1995
0-19-963301-0 Hardback   £65.00
0-19-963300-2 Paperback   £35.95

Green, A.
An introduction to health planning in developing countries
Oxford UP 384pp 2e. Paperback 1999
0-19-262984-0   £25.95

Guerrant, R.L.
Essentials of tropical infectious diseases
Churchill Liv 600pp Paperback 2000
0-443-07909-9   £55.00

Guerrant, R.L.
Tropical infectious diseases
2 vols Churchill Liv 1200pp Hardback 1999
0-443-07908-0   £199.00

Harries, J.R.
Clinical problems in tropical medicine
W B Saunders 236pp Paperback 1998
0-7020-2444-9   £21.95

Hendrickse, R.G.
Paediatrics in the Tropics
Blackwell Science UK 1000pp Hardback 1991
0-632-02675-8   £125.00

Klein, S.
A book for midwives
Macmillan Education 528pp Paperback 1995
0-333-66059-5   £12.25

Markell, E.K.
Medical parasitology
W B Saunders 544pp 8e. Hardback 1998
0-7216-7634-0   £39.00

Nutman, T.B.
Lymphatic filariasis
Imperial College Pr 292pp Paperback 1999
1-86094-059-5   £30.00

Pande, J.N.
Respiratory medicine in the tropics
Oxford UP India 544pp Paperback 2000
0-19-565202-9   £19.95

Peters, W.
Color atlas of tropical medicine parasitology
Mosby 254pp 4e. Hardback 1995
0-7234-2069-6   £34.00

Rozendaal, J.A.
**Vector control: methods for use by individuals
and communities**
WHO 412pp Paperback 1997
92-4-154494-5   £85.00

Sandford-Smith, J.
Eye diseases in hot climates
Butterworth-Heinemann 288pp 3e. Paperback 1997
0-7506-2544-9   £50.00

Savage-King, F.
Nutrition for developing countries
Oxford UP 476pp Paperback 1993
0-19-262233-1   £24.95

Schull, C.R.
Common medical problems in the Tropics
Macmillan Heinemann 533pp 2e. Paperback 1999
0-333-67999-7   £17.25

Stevenson, D.
**Davey and Lightbody's control of disease in the
tropics**
Stanley Thornes 400pp 6e. Paperback 1999
0-412-62740-X   £24.99

Strickland, G.T.
Hunter's tropical medicine
W B Saunders 1232pp 8e. Hardback 1999
0-7216-6223-4   £139.00

Watters, D.A.K.
**Care of the critically ill patient in the Tropics and
Sub-tropics**
Macmillan Heinemann 464pp Paperback 1991
0-333-53799-8   £16.99

Watters, D.A.K.
Gastroenterology in the tropics and subtropics
Macmillan Education 448pp Paperback 1995
0-333-59343-X   £30.95

Werner, D.
Where there is no doctor
Macmillan Heinemann 512pp Paperback 1993
0-333-51651-6   £7.75

Werner, D.
**Where there is no doctor: a village health care
handbook for Africa**
Macmillan Education 500pp Paperback 1994
0-333-51652-4   £7.99

Willan, J.
**Hospital management in the tropics and
subtropics**
Macmillan Education 448pp Paperback 1990
0-333-52257-5   £16.99

World Health Organization
Basic tests for drugs
WHO 91pp Paperback 1998
92-4-154513-5   £16.25

World Health Organization
Care in normal birth
WHO 54pp Paperback 1997
0-11-951748-5   £6.25

World Health Organization
Malaria: a manual for community health workers
WHO 46pp Paperback 1996
92-4-154491-0   £10.00

UROLOGY & NEPHROLOGY

Blandy, J.
Lecture notes on urology
Blackwell Science UK 304pp Paperback 1998
0-632-04202-8   £22.95

Blandy, J.
Transurethral resection
Isis Medical Media 200pp 4e. Hardback 1998
1-899066-84-5   £49.95

Blandy, J.P.
Urology
Blackwell Science UK 648pp 2e. Hardback 1995
0-632-03679-6   £110.00

Brenner, B.M.
The kidney
2 vols W B Saunders 2880pp 6e. Hardback 1999
0-7216-7998-6   £265.00

Brumfitt, W.
Urinary tract infections
Arnold 368pp Hardback 1998
0-412-63050-8   £90.00

Bullock, N.
Essential urology
Churchill Liv 369pp 2e. Paperback 1994
0-443-04807-X   £24.95

Cameron, J.S.
Kidney failure: the facts
Oxford Paperbacks 248pp Paperback 1996
0-19-262643-4   £11.99

Cardozo, L.
Urinary incontinence in primary care
Isis Medical Media 128pp Paperback 2000
1-901865-68-1   £25.00

Cattell, W.R.
Infections of the kidney and urinary tract
Oxford UP 360pp Hardback 1996
0-19-262441-5 £69.50

Coptcoat, M.J.
Laparoscopy in urology
Blackwell Science UK 168pp Hardback 1994
0-86542-814-X £59.50

Davison, A.M.
Oxford textbook of clinical nephrology
Oxford UP 3248pp 2e. 1997
0-19-262413-X Hardback £350.00
0-19-268581-3 CD-ROM £293.75

Dawson, C.
ABC of urology
BMJ Books 60pp Paperback 1997
0-7279-1075-2 £14.95

Jamison, R.
Textbook of nephrology
Arnold 1172pp Hardback 1997
0-412-60930-4 £145.00

Johnson, R.
Comprehensive clinical nephrology
Mosby 1068pp Hardback 2000
0-7234-3117-5 £149.00

Kirby, R.
Erectile dysfunction
Isis Medical Media 120pp Paperback 1999
1-901865-24-X £19.95

Kirby, R.
Men's health
Isis Medical Media 300pp Paperback 1999
1-899066-92-6 £39.95

Kirby, R.
Shared care for prostatic diseases
Isis Medical Media 165pp Paperback 2000
1-901865-60-6 £22.50

Lloyd-Davies, W.
A colour atlas of urology
Mosby 288pp 2e. Hardback 1993
0-7234-1912-4 £65.00

Lote, C.J.
Principles of renal physiology
Kluwer Academic Publ 224pp 4e. Paperback 2000
0-7923-6178-4 £13.95

Mellon, J.K.
Synopses in urology
Blackwell Science UK 168pp Paperback 1998
0-632-05072-1 £15.95

Mundy, A.R.
The scientific basis of urology
Isis Medical Media 544pp Hardback 1999
1-899066-21-7 £99.95

Schrier, R.W.
Renal and electrolyte disorders
Williams and Wilkins 784pp 5e. Paperback 1997
0-316-77454-5 £42.50

Tanagho, E.A.
Smith's general urology
Appleton and Lange 775pp 15e. Paperback 2000
0-8385-8607-4 £29.99

Walsh, P.C.
Campbell's urology
3 vols W B Saunders 3840pp 7e. Hardback 1997
0-7216-4461-9 £299.00

Whitfield, H.
Textbook of genito-urinary surgery
2 vols Blackwell Science UK 2112pp 2e.
Hardback 1998
0-632-03774-1 £395.00

Williams, G.
Color atlas of renal diseases
Mosby 385pp 2e. Hardback 1993
0-7234-1719-9 £60.00

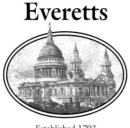
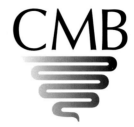

JOURNALS

Critical Care Medicine & New Horizons
monthly
Williams & Wilkins £274.71

ACCIDENT & EMERGENCY MEDICINE

Annals of Emergency Medicine
monthly
Mosby £190.08

Injury - International Journal for the Care of the Injured
monthly
Elsevier Science £374.70

Emergency Medicine Journal
bi-monthly
BMJ Publishing £199.00

Journal of Trauma - Injury Infection and Critical Care
monthly
Williams & Wilkins £275.43

AIDS & HIV

AIDS - an International Monthly Journal
monthly
Williams & Wilkins £850.69

AIDS Care - Psychological and Socio-Medical Aspects of AIDS HIV
bi-monthly
Taylor & Francis £460.00

International Journal of STD and AIDS
monthly
Royal Society of Medicine £236.00

AIDS Research and Human Retroviruses
monthly
Mary Ann Liebert £948.95

ANAESTHESIA & INTENSIVE CARE

Anaesthesia
monthly
Blackwell Science £294.00

Anesthesiology - Hagerstown
monthly
Williams & Wilkins £313.74

British Journal of Anaesthesia
monthly
Oxford UP £230.00

ANATOMY & HISTOLOGY

Developmental Dynamics
monthly
Wiley £1,800.04

Histopathology
monthly
Blackwell Science £427.00

Journal of Anatomy
bi-monthly
Cambridge UP £576.00

Journal of Histochemistry and Cytochemistry
monthly
Histochemical Society £419.60

BIOCHEMICAL & CELL BIOLOGY

Biochemical Journal & Biochemical Journal Reviews
bi-monthly
Portland Press £1,185.00

EMBO Journal - European Molecular Biology Organization
bi-monthly
Oxford UP £795.00

Cell
bi-monthly
Cell Press £604.66

Journal of Biological Chemistry
weekly
Journal of Biological Chemistry £1,477.58

CARDIOLOGY

American Heart Journal
monthly
Mosby £281.17

American Journal of Cardiology
bi-monthly
Reed Elsevier £305.56

Cardiovascular Research
monthly
Elsevier Science £460.20

Circulation - Hagertown
weekly
Williams & Wilkins   £483.44

Evidence Based Cardiovascular Medicine
quarterly
Harcourt   £170.00

Heart - London
monthly
BMJ Publishing   £300.00

Journal of the American College of Cardiology
monthly
Elsevier Science   £246.74

Journal of Thoracic and Cardiovascular Surgery
monthly
Mosby   £302.69

COMMUNITY CARE

Community Care
weekly
Quadrant Subscriptions   £72.00

Health and Social Care in the Community
bi-monthly
Blackwell Science   £281.00

COMPLEMENTARY MEDICINE

Alternative and Complementary Therapies
bi-monthly
Mary Ann Liebert   £195.81

British Homeopathic Journal
quarterly
Macmillan   £110.00

Complementary Therapies in Medicine
quarterly
Harcourt   £160.00

Journal of Alternative and Complementary Medicine - New York
bi-monthly
Mary Ann Liebert   £175.02

COMPUTING

British Journal of Healthcare Computing and Information Management
monthly
BJHC Ltd.   £55.00

DENTISTRY & ORAL MEDICINE

British Dental Journal & Dental Business
weekly
Macmillan   £367.00

British Journal of Oral and Maxillofacial Surgery
bi-monthly
Harcourt   £252.00

Journal of the American Dental Association
monthly
American Dental Association   £109.75

Journal of Dental Research & Special Issues & Advances in Dental Research & Abstracts
monthly
American and Inter Association for
Dental Research   £258.22

DERMATOLOGY

Archives of Dermatology
monthly
American Medical Association   £295.00

British Journal of Dermatology & Supplements
monthly
Blackwell Science   £520.00

Clinical and Experimental Dermatology
bi-monthly
Blackwell Science   £509.00

Journal of the American Academy of Dermatology
monthly
Mosby   £294.80

EAR NOSE & THROAT

Archives of Otolaryngology - Head and Neck Surgery
monthly
American Medical Association   £295.00

Clinical Otolaryngology and Allied Sciences
bi-monthly
Blackwell Science   £420.00

Journal of Laryngology and Otology & Supplements
monthly
Royal Society of Medicine   £150.00

Laryngoscope
monthly
Williams & Wilkins   £252.47

ENDOCRINOLOGY, METABOLISM & DIABETES

Bailliere's Best Practice and Research In Clinical Endocrinology and Metabolism
quarterly
Harcourt   £176.00

Clinical Endocrinology - Oxford
monthly
Blackwell Science   £582.00

Diabetes - American Diabetes Association
monthly
American Diabetic Association   £272.56

Diabetic Medicine
monthly
Blackwell Science   £437.00

Endocrinology
monthly
Endocrine Society   £512.13

Journal of Clinical Endocrinology and Metabolism
monthly
Endocrine Society   £370.11

Journal of Endocrinology
monthly
Society for Endocrinology   £430.00

EVIDENCE-BASED MEDICINE

Bandolier
monthly
Hayward Medical Communications   £38.88

British Journal of Clinical Governance
quarterly
MCB University Press   £199.00

Clinical Evidence
bi-annually
BMJ Publishing   £160.00

Cochrane Library LAN-1-5 Users CD-ROM
quarterly
Update Software Ltd.   £270.00

Effective Health Care
bi-monthly
Royal Society of Medicine   £78.00

Evidence Based Health Care
quarterly
Harcourt   £170.00

Evidence Based Medicine
bi-monthly
BMJ Publishing   £120.00

Journal of Evaluation in Clinical Practice
quarterly
Blackwell Science   £323.00

FORENSIC MEDICINE

American Journal of Forensic Medicine and Pathology
quarterly
Williams & Wilkins   £322.77

Journal of Forensic Sciences
bi-monthly
American Society for Testing & Materials   £196.53

Medicine Science and the Law
quarterly
Chiltern Publishers   £69.00

Medico Legal Journal
quarterly
CLT Professional Publishing   £80.00

GASTROENTEROLOGY

Bailliere's Best Practice and Research in Clinical Gastroenterology
bi-monthly
Harcourt   £214.00

Gastroenterology - Orlando
monthly
WB Saunders   £442.56

Gut
monthly
BMJ Publishing   £300.00

Hepatology
monthly
WB Saunders   £550.86

GENERAL & BIBLIOGRAPHIES

Bulletin of the Medical Library Association
quarterly
Medical Library Association   £134.79

Current Serials Received
annual
Turpin   £95.00

Health Information and Libraries Journal
quarterly
Blackwell Science £195.00

Nature
weekly
Macmillan £370.00

New Scientist - UK Edition
weekly
Quadrant Subscriptions £97.00

Science - International Edition - AAAS
weekly
American Association for the Advancement
of Science £327.80

Scientific American
monthly
CDS Communications £43.03

GENERAL PRACTICE

**British Journal of General Practice - Journal of
the Royal College of General Practitioners**
monthly
World Wide Subscription Services £130.00

Education for General Practice
quarterly
Radcliffe Medical £120.00

Family Practice
bi-monthly
Oxford UP £175.00

Journal of Family Practice
monthly
Dowden Publishing Co. £190.08

Practitioner - London
monthly
Miller Freeman £74.50

GENETICS

American Journal of Human Genetics
monthly
University of Chicago Press £455.47

Journal of Medical Genetics
monthly
BMJ Publishing £284.00

Nature Genetics
monthly
Macmillan £520.00

GERIATRIC MEDICINE

Age and Ageing
bi-monthly
Oxford UP £180.00

Geriatric Medicine - Sevenoaks
monthly
Inside Communications £69.00

Geriatrics - Duluth
monthly
Advanstar Communications £86.08

Journal of the American Geriatrics Society
monthly
Williams & Wilkins £294.09

**Journals of Gerontology - A & Journals of
Gerontology - B**
monthly
Gerontological Society of America £463.36

HAEMATOLOGY

**Bailliere's Best Practice and Research in Clinical
Haematology**
quarterly
Harcourt £163.00

Blood
bi-monthly
WB Saunders £701.49

British Journal of Haematology
monthly
Blackwell Science £566.00

HEALTH ADMINISTRATION

British Journal of Healthcare Management
monthly
Mark Allen Publishing £200.00

Clinician in Management
quarterly
British Association of Medical Managers £129.60

Health Service Abstracts
monthly
Dept of Health Library £40.00

Health Service Journal
weekly
EMAP Readerlink £85.00

Health Services Management Research
quarterly
Royal Society of Medicine   £110.00

NHS Magazine
quarterly
Atlas Public Relations Ltd   £17.28

Quality in Health Care
quarterly
BMJ Publishing   £155.52

HEALTH PROMOTION

Health Education Journal
quarterly
Royal Society of Medicine   £63.00

Health Promotion International
quarterly
Oxford UP   £148.50

IMMUNOLOGY & ALLERGY

Clinical and Experimental Immunology
monthly
Blackwell Science   £768.00

Immunity
monthly
Cell Press   £451.88

Immunology
monthly
Blackwell Science   £546.00

Journal of Allergy and Clinical Immunology
monthly
Mosby   £283.32

Journal of Immunology
bi-monthly
Journal of Immunology   £454.75

Nature Immunology
monthly
Macmillan   £395.00

INFECTIOUS DISEASES

Infection and Immunity
monthly
American Society for Microbiology   £466.23

Journal of Infectious Diseases
monthly
University of Chicago Press   £301.98

Journal of Hospital Infection
monthly
Harcourt   £371.00

Journal of Infection
bi-monthly
Harcourt   £279.00

MEDICAL ETHICS

Journal of Medical Ethics & Medical Humanities
bi-monthly
BMJ Publishing   £160.00

MEDICINE

American Journal of Medicine
monthly
American Journal of Medicine   £284.75

Annals of Internal Medicine - Including Index
bi-monthly
American College of Physicians   £230.96

Archives of Internal Medicine
bi-monthly
American Medical Association   £275.00

British Medical Bulletin
quarterly
Royal Society of Medicine   £160.00

BMJ - British Medical Journal - General Practice Edition - UK Subscribers Only
weekly
BMJ Publishing   £255.00

Hospital Medicine - Salisbury
monthly
Mark Allen Publishing   £210.00

JAMA - Journal of the American Medical Association - US Edition
weekly
American Medical Association   £239.90

Journal of Clinical Investigation
bi-monthly
American Society for Clinical Investigation   £491.33

Journal of the Royal College of Physicians of London
bi-monthly
Royal College Physicians   £100.00

Journal of the Royal Society of Medicine & Supplements
monthly
Royal Society of Medicine   £142.00

Lancet - Including Index
weekly
Lancet £365.00

Medical Clinics of North America
bi-monthly
WB Saunders £164.25

Medicine - Baltimore
bi-monthly
Williams & Wilkins £256.78

Medicine - UK Edition
monthly
Medicine Publishing Group £190.00

Nature Medicine
monthly
Macmillan £520.00

New England Journal of Medicine - Unbound Volume
weekly
Medical Publishing Group £265.00

Postgraduate Medical Journal & Supplements
monthly
Professional & Scientific Publications £224.00

QJM - Monthly Journal of the Association of Physicians
monthly
Oxford UP £260.00

Update - Journal of Continuing Education for General Practitioners - UK Ed & Training Update
weekly
Quadrant Subscription Services £102.00

MICROBIOLOGY

Epidemiology and Infection
bi-monthly
Cambridge UP £258.00

Journal of Clinical Microbiology
monthly
American Society for Microbiology £317.03

Journal of Medical Microbiology
monthly
Williams & Wilkins £555.88

NEUROLOGY & NEUROSURGERY

Annals of Neurology
monthly
Williams & Wilkins £336.40

Archives of Neurology
monthly
American Medical Association £295.00

Brain
monthly
Oxford UP £320.00

British Journal of Neurosurgery
bi-monthly
Taylor & Francis £489.00

Journal of Neurology Neurosurgery and Psychiatry
monthly
BMJ Publishing £314.00

Journal of Neurosurgery
monthly
American Association Neurol Surgeons £139.86

Nature Neuroscience
monthly
Macmillan £435.00

Neurology
bi-monthly
Williams & Wilkins £431.80

Neurosurgery - Hagerstown
monthly
Williams & Wilkins £363.65

NUTRITION & DIETETICS

American Journal of Clinical Nutrition
monthly
American Society for Clinical Nutrition £172.14

British Journal of Nutrition
monthly
CAB International £475.00

Journal of the American Dietetic Association
monthly
American Dietetic Association £147.04

Journal of Human Nutrition and Dietetics
bi-monthly
Blackwell Science £235.00

OBSTETRICS & GYNAECOLOGY

American Journal of Obstetrics and Gynecology
monthly
Mosby £294.80

Bailliere's Best Practice and Research in Clinical Obstetrics and Gynaecology
bi-monthly
Harcourt £216.00

British Journal of Obstetrics and Gynaecology & Supplements
monthly
Blackwell Science £168.42

Contemporary Reviews in Obstetrics and Gynecology
quarterly
Parthenon £120.00

Current Opinion in Obstetrics and Gynecology
bi-monthly
Williams & Wilkins £402.39

Evidence Based Obstetrics and Gynaecology
quarterly
Harcourt £170.00

Fertility and Sterility
monthly
Elsevier Science £221.20

Journal of Obstetrics and Gynaecology - Abingdon
bi-monthly
Taylor & Francis £215.00

Obstetrics and Gynecology - New York
monthly
Elsevier Science £259.65

OCCUPATIONAL THERAPY

American Journal of Occupational Therapy
bi-monthly
American Occup Therapy Association £93.25

Australian Occupational Therapy Journal
quarterly
Blackwell Science £132.69

British Journal of Occupational Therapy
monthly
College Occup Therapists £96.00

British Journal of Therapy and Rehabilitation
monthly
Mark Allen Publishing £175.00

Canadian Journal of Occupational Therapy
bi-monthly
Canadian Association Occ Therapists £45.08

Journal of Occupational Science - Australia
quarterly
Univ. South Adelaide £37.07

Occupational Therapy International
quarterly
Turpin £120.00

Occupational Therapy in Health Care
quarterly
Haworth £182.01

Occupational Therapy in Mental Health
quarterly
Haworth £286.01

ONCOLOGY

British Journal of Cancer & Supplements
bi-monthly
Harcourt £900.00

Cancer & Cancer Cytopathology
weekly
Wiley £469.81

Cancer Research & Clinical Cancer Research & Proceedings American Association of Cancer Research
weekly
American Association of Cancer Research £898.59

Journal of Clinical Oncology
bi-monthly
Williams & Wilkins £416.74

Journal of the National Cancer Institute & Monographs
bi-monthly
Oxford UP £232.00

OPHTHALMOLOGY

American Journal of Ophthalmology
monthly
Ophthalmic Publishing £297.67

Archives of Ophthalmology - Chicago
monthly
American Medical Association £275.00

British Journal of Ophthalmology
monthly
BMJ Publishing £333.00

Eye - An International Journal of Ophthalmology
bi-monthly
Royal College of Ophthalmologists £257.00

Ophthalmology
monthly
Kable Fulfillment Service £317.76

ORTHOPAEDICS

Acta Orthopaedica Scandinavica & Supplements
monthly
Taylor & Francis £145.00

Clinical Orthopaedics and Related Research
monthly
Williams & Wilkins   £550.14

Current Orthopaedics
bi-monthly
Harcourt   £327.00

Journal of Bone and Joint Surgery - Combined Edition American & British Volumes
bi-monthly
British Editorial Society of Bone and Joint Surgery
                                                     £196.00

Journal of Pediatric Orthopaedics
bi-monthly
Williams & Wilkins   £379.44

Orthopedic Clinics of North America
quarterly
W B Saunders   £185.06

PAEDIATRICS

Acta Paediatrica - International Journal of Paediatrics & Supplements
monthly
Taylor & Francis   £300.00

Archives of Pediatrics and Adolescent Medicine
monthly
American Medical Association   £275.00

Archives of Disease in Childhood & Fetal and Neonatal Edition
monthly
BMJ Publishing   £323.00

Journal of Pediatrics
monthly
Mosby   £281.17

Journal of Pediatric Surgery
monthly
WB Saunders   £357.91

Pediatric Clinics of North America
bi-monthly
WB Saunders   £167.13

Pediatrics - English Edition
monthly
American Acad Pediatrics   £154.21

PALLIATIVE MEDICINE

European Journal of Palliative Care - English Edition
bi-monthly
Hayward Medical Communications   £205.20

Palliative Medicine
bi-monthly
Edward Arnold   £352.00

PATHOLOGY & LABORATORY MEDICINE

American Journal of Clinical Pathology
monthly
American Soc Clin Pathologists   £326.36

American Journal of Pathology & Journal of Molecular Diagnostics
monthly
Jnl. of Pathology   £344.29

Archives of Pathology and Laboratory Medicine
monthly
College of American Pathologists   £164.98

Clinical Chemistry
monthly
American Association for Clinical Chemistry   £510.69

Journal of Clinical Pathology & Molecular Pathology
monthly
BMJ Publishing   £407.00

Journal of Laboratory and Clinical Medicine
monthly
Mosby   £286.20

Journal of Pathology
monthly
Wiley   £767.48

Laboratory Investigation
monthly
Williams & Wilkins   £388.04

PHARMACOLOGY & THERAPEUTICS

Adverse Drug Reaction Bulletin - Andover
bi-monthly
Williams & Wilkins   £68.86

British Journal of Clinical Pharmacology
monthly
Blackwell Science   £510.00

Clinical Pharmacology and Therapeutics
monthly
Mosby   £281.89

Drug and Therapeutics Bulletin - English Edition & Treatment Notes
bi-monthly
Consumers Association   £49.00

Journal of Pharmacy and Pharmacology
bi-monthly
Pharmaceutical Press   £520.00

PHYSIOLOGY

Journal of Applied Physiology
monthly
American Physiological Soc.   £670.64

Journal of Physiology & Cumulative Author and Subject Index
bi-monthly
Cambridge UP   £1,448.00

PHYSIOTHERAPY

Archives of Physical Medicine and Rehabilitation
monthly
W B Saunders   £238.85

Australian Journal of Physiotherapy
quarterly
Australian Physiotherapy Association   £42.92

Journal of Manual and Manipulative Therapy
quarterly
JMMT   £107.59

Manual Therapy
quarterly
Harcourt   £165.00

Physical Therapy
monthly
American Physiol Ther Association   £86.08

Physical Therapy Reviews
quarterly
Maney Publishing   £144.00

Physiotherapy - Journal of the Chartered Society of Physiotherapy
monthly
Chartered Society of Physiotherapy   £120.00

Physiotherapy Research International
quarterly
Turpin   £120.00

Physiotherapy Theory and Practice
quarterly
Taylor & Francis   £183.00

PLASTIC SURGERY

British Journal of Plastic Surgery
bi-monthly
Harcourt   £217.00

Burns - the Journal of the International Society for Burn Injuries
bi-monthly
Elsevier Science   £366.09

Journal of Hand Surgery - American Volume
bi-monthly
WB Saunders   £248.18

Journal of Hand Surgery - British and European Volume
bi-monthly
Harcourt   £240.00

Plastic and Reconstructive Surgery - Baltimore
monthly
Williams & Wilkins   £415.30

PODIATRY

Podiatry Now & British Journal of Podiatry
monthly
Society of Chiropodists   £59.40

Clinics in Podiatric Medicine and Surgery
quarterly
W B Saunders   £169.99

Foot - Sidcup
quarterly
Harcourt   £156.00

Journal of the American Podiatric Medical Association
monthly
American Pod Medical Association   £98.98

PSYCHIATRY & PSYCHOLOGY

Acta Psychiatrica Scandinavica & Supplements
monthly
Munksgaard   £331.21

Advances in Psychiatric Treatment
bi-monthly
Royal Society of Medicine   £88.00

American Journal of Psychiatry
monthly
American Psych Publishing   £290.50

Archives of General Psychiatry
monthly
American Medical Association £275.00

British Journal of Clinical Psychology
quarterly
Turpin £145.00

British Journal of Medical Psychology
quarterly
Turpin £144.00

British Journal of Psychiatry
monthly
Royal Society of Medicine £209.00

Evidence Based Mental Health
quarterly
BMJ Publishing £141.48

Journal of Child Psychology and Psychiatry and Allied Disciplines
bi-monthly
Cambridge UP £232.00

Psychiatric Bulletin
monthly
Royal Society of Medicine £64.00

Psychological Bulletin
bi-monthly
American Psychol Association £275.43

Psychological Medicine
bi-monthly
Cambridge UP £266.00

PUBLIC HEALTH & EPIDEMIOLOGY

American Journal of Epidemiology & Epidemiologic Reviews
bi-monthly
Oxford UP £215.00

American Journal of Public Health
monthly
American Public Health Association £171.07

Health Statistics Quarterly
quarterly
Stationery Office £81.00

International Journal of Epidemiology
bi-monthly
Oxford UP £247.00

Journal of Epidemiology and Community Health
monthly
BMJ Publishing £247.00

Journal of Public Health Medicine
quarterly
Oxford UP £155.00

Occupational and Environmental Medicine
monthly
BMJ Publishing £212.00

Population Trends
quarterly
Stationery Office £81.00

Public Health
bi-monthly
Macmillan £170.00

RADIOLOGY & RADIOGRAPHY

AJR - American Journal of Roentgenology
monthly
American Roentgen Ray Soc £204.42

British Journal of Radiology
monthly
British Institute of Radiology £360.00

Clinical Radiology
monthly
Harcourt £310.00

Radiography - Sidcup
quarterly
Harcourt £143.00

Radiology & RSNA Index to Imaging Literature & RSNA Scientific Program
monthly
Association of University Radiologists £193.66

RESPIRATORY MEDICINE

American Journal of Respiratory and Critical Care Medicine
monthly
American Thoracic Society £222.36

Chest & Supplements
monthly
American College Chest Physicians £150.63

Respiratory Medicine
monthly
Harcourt £290.00

Thorax
monthly
BMJ Publishing £292.00

RHEUMATOLOGY

Annals of the Rheumatic Diseases
monthly
BMJ Publishing   £336.00

Arthritis and Rheumatism & Supplements, & Arthritis Care and Research x 20
Williams & Wilkins   £326.13

Bailliere's Best Practice and Research in Clinical Rheumatology
quarterly
Harcourt   £184.00

Journal of Rheumatology & Supplements
monthly
Journal of Rheumatology   £186.49

Rheumatology - Oxford & Supplements
monthly
Oxford UP   £350.00

SEXUALLY TRANSMITTED DISEASES

Sexually Transmitted Diseases
monthly
Williams & Wilkins   £274.00

Sexually Transmitted Infections
bi-monthly
BMJ Publishing   £199.00

SPEECH THERAPY

ASHA Leader
bi-monthly
American Speech-Language-Hearing
Association   £107.59

International Journal of Language and Communication Disorders
quarterly
Taylor & Francis   £191.00

Journal of Speech Language and Hearing Research
bi-monthly
American Speech-Language-Hearing Assn.   £218.77

SPORTS MEDICINE

American Journal of Sports Medicine
bi-monthly
Journal of Sports Medicine   £86.08

British Journal of Sports Medicine
bi-monthly
BMJ Publishing   £199.00

Medicine and Science in Sports and Exercise
monthly
Williams & Wilkins   £342.14

Sports Medicine - ADIS International
monthly
Adis International   £570.23

SUBSTANCE ABUSE

Addiction
monthly
Taylor & Francis   £650.00

Alcohol and Alcoholism
bi-monthly
Oxford UP   £340.00

Journal of Studies on Alcohol & Supplements
bi-monthly
Alcohol Research Document   £136.28

SURGERY

American Journal of Surgery
monthly
Reed Elsevier   £254.63

Annals of the Royal College of Surgeons of England & Bulletin
monthly
Royal Society of Medicine   £110.00

Annals of Surgery
monthly
Williams & Wilkins   £369.39

Archives of Surgery
monthly
American Medical Association   £275.00

British Journal of Surgery
monthly
Blackwell Science   £146.00

Journal of the American College of Surgeons
monthly
Elsevier Science   £228.80

Surgery - St Louis
monthly
Mosby   £268.97

Surgery - Oxford
monthly
Medicine Group   £190.00

Surgical Clinics of North America
bi-monthly
W B Saunders £192.95

TROPICAL MEDICINE

American Journal of Tropical Medicine and Hygiene & Tropical Medicine and Hygiene News
monthly
Allen Press £322.77

Annals of Tropical Medicine and Parasitology
bi-monthly
Taylor & Francis £389.00

Annals of Tropical Paediatrics
quarterly
Taylor & Francis £298.00

Bulletin of the World Health Organization
monthly
World Health Organisation £83.78

Journal of Tropical Pediatrics
bi-monthly
Oxford UP £160.00

Transactions of the Royal Society of Tropical Medicine and Hygiene
bi-monthly
Royal Society of Tropical Medicine £155.00

Tropical Diseases Bulletin
monthly
CAB International £284.00

Tropical Doctor
quarterly
Royal Society of Medicine £47.00

Tropical Medicine and International Health
monthly
Blackwell Science £416.00

UROLOGY & NEPHROLOGY

BJU International - British Journal of Urology - Including Free CD ROM & Supplements
bi-monthly
Blackwell Science £273.00

Journal of Urology
monthly
Williams & Wilkins £447.58

Kidney International & Kidney International - Supplements
monthly
Blackwell Science £753.14

Nephrology Dialysis Transplantation
monthly
Oxford UP £410.00

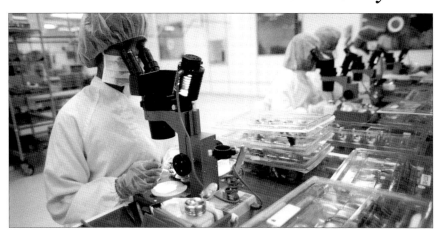
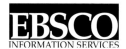

AUTHOR INDEX

O

Oatley K. 60
O'Brien E. 6
O'Dowd T. 23
Ogden J. 60
Ogilvie C. 12
Oh T.E. 3
Olson K.R. 53
O'Neill P.A. 37
Otto C.M. 6
Ovretveit J. 8, 29

P

Page C. 54
Page S.R. 17
Palastanga N. 55
Palfreeman A. 2
Pallen M. 9
Pallister C. 50
Palmer K.T. 23
Palmer M. 35
Palmer S. 10
Pande J.N. 72
Parfitt K. 54
Park G. 39
Parkes C.M. 49
Parkes W.R. 61
Parkin A.J. 60
Parkinson J. 16
Parsley K. 29
Parums D.V. 50
Patel P.R. 63
Paterson A. 63
Paterson-Brown S. 70
Pathy M.S.J. 25
Paton C. 27
Patten J.P. 39
Payne R.A. 10
Payne S.D.W. 68
Payne-James J. 40
Peakman M. 30
Peat M. 64
Peckham M. 44
Pedretti L.W. 43
Penneys N.S. 2
Penson J. 49
Perkin G.D. 39
Perkins A.C. 63
Perkins R. 8
Peters W. 72
Petrie A. 18
Phelan P.D. 48
Phillips A.F. 20
Phillips A.J. 45
Phillips R.K.S. 21
Philp I. 25
Philps J.W. 57
Pickles B. 55
Pickup J.C. 17
Pike S. 29
Pine C. 11

Pinnock C. 3
Pitt-Brooke J. 64
Pizzo P.A. 2
Playfair J.H.L. 30
Po A.L.W. 19
Pocock G. 54
Polden M. 55
Pollard S. 27
Pollock D.J. 70
Pollock R.E. 44
Polnay L. 48
Ponsford J. 64
Pope C. 36
Porter M. 60
Porter R. 16
Poston G.J. 70
Pounder R.E. 12, 21
Powell M.A. 29
Powers M. 20
Price S. 8
Pringle M. 23
Provan D. 26
Prowle M. 26
Pryor J.A. 55
Prys-Roberts C. 3
Punwar A. 43
Puri B.K. 59

Q

Quarini C.A. 16
Quick C. 70

R

Rainsbury P.A. 31
Ramrakha P.S. 1
Ranade W. 27
Rang H.P. 54
Ray K.K. 63
Read M. 68
Redford J.B. 57
Reece D. 16
Reed A. 55
Reed K. 43
Rees J. 65
Rees L. 59
Reeves G. 30
Reid J.L. 54
Rhee D.J. 45
Rhodes J.M. 21
Richards P. 16
Richardson M. 38
Ridsdale L. 19
Riley J. 28
Rimoin D.L. 24
Rintoul R.F. 70
Ritter J.M. 54
Ritter S. 8
Robbins J. 49
Robbins M. 23, 49
Roberton N.R.C. 48
Roberts G.M. 63

Roberts K. 28
Robertson J.R. 68
Robinson M.J. 48
Robson P 68.
Rock J.A. 41
Rockwood C.A. 46
Roitt I. 30
Roitt I.M. 30
Rosai J. 50
Rose J. 57
Rosenberg R.N. 39
Roses D.F. 44
Rowe F.J. 45
Rowland L.P. 39
Rowlands B. 9
Rowlands S. 23
Roy F.H. 45
Royal College of
  Obstetricians and
  Gynaecologists 31
Royal Commission on
  Long Term Care 25
Rozendaal J.A. 72
Rubenstein D. 37
Rubin E. 50
Rubin P.C. 41
Rushman G.B. 3
Russell A.D. 31
Russell J.A. 65
Russell R. 41
Russell R.C.G. 70
Rustin L. 67
Rutter S.M. 59
Ryan M. 32
Rycroft R.J.G. 12

S

Sabiston Jr D.C. 70
Sackett D. 18, 19
Sadler T. 4
Saffar P. 56
Salter B. 27
Sambandan S. 23
Sande. M.A. 2
Sandford-Smith J. 72
Sarafino E.P. 60
Sasada M. 3
Saunders C. 49
Savage-King F. 72
Savin A. 12
Scally P. 63
Scambler G.B.P 61.
Schoub 2
Schoub B.D. 2
Schrier R. 25
Schrier R.W. 73
Schull C.R. 72
Schwartz S.I. 70
Scotland A. 29
Scott D. 29
Scott N.A. 12
Scratcherd T. 54

Scriven A. 29
Scriver C.R. 17
Scrutton S. 10
Scully C. 11
Seaton A. 61, 65
Seedhouse D. 29, 35
Seibel M. 31
Settle J. 56
Shanson D.C. 38
Shapiro L.M. 6
Sharif K.W. 41
Sharkey P. 8
Sharp P.F. 63
Shaw R.W. 41
Shaw V. 40
Shearman D.J.C. 21
Shepherd R. 56
Sherlock S. 21
Sherry E. 68
Shils M.E. 40
Shipley M. 66
Shukla R.B. 25
Shulman S.T. 31
Sidell M. 29
Silagy C. 19
Silverman J. 7
Simnett I. 29
Simnett K.I. 29
Simonds A.K. 65
Sims A. 59
Sinclair A.J. 25
Sinclair D. 48
Singer M. 3
Singer R. 23
Singleton J. 35
Sinnatamby C.S. 4
Skeel R.T. 44
Skinner D. 1
Skinner D.V. 1
Slade R. 41
Sleigh J.D. 38
Smith A.F. 50
Smith B.G.N. 11
Smith C. 26
Smith J. 28
Smith J.M.B. 70
Smith P.C. 26
Smith T. 16, 35
Snaith M.L. 66
Snashall D. 61
Snell R.S. 4, 45
Snowling M. 67
Soames J.V. 11
Society for the Study of
  Addiction 68
Solomon L. 46
Sonnex C. 66
Soothill K. 28
Souhami R.L. 37, 44
Southgate L. 31
Spalton D.J. 45
Spector T.D. 53
Speight T.M. 54